Practices of Traditionalization in Central Asia

Practices of Traditionalization in Central Asia focuses on how tradition is 'everyday-ified' in contemporary Central Asia, including Tatarstan and Tibet, and what people seek to achieve in its name. The case studies range from political demonstrations and industrial workers' gatherings to institutions of religious education, minority communities, weddings, and the Internet.

In this volume, we regard tradition as a practice that needs to be explored in its institutional and interactional context at a particular time, rather than as a reliable guide to the past: tradition can only be judged from the present; it is an interpretative concept, not a descriptive one. While the scholarly debate has so far centered on what tradition entails and what it does not, including the question of invention and ownership, less attention has been devoted to investigating how tradition is enacted, enforced, or motivated – in short, how it 'gets done.' In Central Asia, practices of traditionalization are closely related to the transformation of the socialist order and the emergence of highly stratified societies. This volume asks the following: When does tradition emerge as a line of argumentation, who are the actors invoking it, and how is it being (materially) manifested?

Practices of Traditionalization in Central Asia will be of great interest to scholars of Central Asia, Anthropology, History, Political Science, and Sociology.

The chapters were originally published as a special issue of *Central Asian Survey*.

Judith Beyer specializes in political and legal anthropology. She conducts long-term ethnographic fieldwork in Central Asia (Kyrgyzstan) and Southeast Asia (Myanmar) and increasingly in Europe.

Peter Finke specializes in economic anthropology, political economy, and post-socialist transformations. He has worked on pastoral nomadism, identity, cognitive anthropology, and norms and ideologies in Mongolia and Central Asia where he carried out extensive field research.

Central Asian Studies

27 Growing Up in the North Caucasus
Society, Family, Religion and Education
Irina Molodikova and Alan Watt

28 Soviet Orientalism and the Creation of Central Asian Nations
Alfrid K. Bustanov

29 Soviet Nation-Building in Central Asia
The Making of the Kazakh and Uzbek Nations
Grigol Ubiria

30 The Afghan-Central Asia Borderland
The State and Local Leaders
Suzanne Levi-Sanchez

31 Kyrgyzstan – Regime Security and Foreign Policy
Kemel Toktomushev

32 Legal Pluralism in Central Asia
Local Jurisdiction and Customary Practices
Mahabat Sadyrbek

33 Identity, History and Trans-Nationality in Central Asia
The Mountain Communities of Pamir
Edited by Carole Faucher and Dagikhudo Dagiev

34 Critical Approaches to Security in Central Asia
Edited by Edward Lemon

35 Russian Practices of Governance in Eurasia
Frontier Power Dynamics, 16–19th Century
Gulnar T. Kendirbai

36 Practices of Traditionalization in Central Asia
Edited by Judith Beyer and Peter Finke

For more information about this series, please visit: https://www.routledge.com/asianstudies/series/CAS

Practices of Traditionalization in Central Asia

Edited by
Judith Beyer and Peter Finke

Routledge
Taylor & Francis Group
LONDON AND NEW YORK

First published 2020
by Routledge
2 Park Square, Milton Park, Abingdon, Oxon, OX14 4RN

and by Routledge
52 Vanderbilt Avenue, New York, NY 10017

Routledge is an imprint of the Taylor & Francis Group, an informa business

British Library Cataloguing-in-Publication Data
A catalogue record for this book is available from the British Library

ISBN13: 978-0-367-89396-5

Typeset in Myriad Pro
by codeMantra

Publisher's Note
The publisher accepts responsibility for any inconsistencies that may have arisen during the conversion of this book from journal articles to book chapters, namely the inclusion of journal terminology.

Contents

Citation Information

The chapters in this book were originally published in the *Central Asian Survey*, volume 38, issue 3 (September 2019). When citing this material, please use the original page numbering for each article, as follows:

Introduction
Practices of traditionalization in Central Asia
Judith Beyer and Peter Finke
Central Asian Survey, volume 38, issue 3 (September 2019), pp. 310–328

Chapter 1
Women of protest, men of applause: political activism, gender and tradition in Kyrgyzstan
Judith Beyer and Aijarkyn Kojobekova
Central Asian Survey, volume 38, issue 3 (September 2019), pp. 329–345

Chapter 2
Traditionalization, or the making of a reputation: women, weddings and expenditure in Tajikistan
Juliette Cleuziou
Central Asian Survey, volume 38, issue 3 (September 2019), pp. 346–362

Chapter 3
The body global and the body traditional: a digital ethnography of Instagram and nationalism in Kazakhstan and Russia
Diana T. Kudaibergenova
Central Asian Survey, volume 38, issue 3 (September 2019), pp. 363–380

Chapter 4
The veterans' gala: the use of tradition in an industrial labour conflict in contemporary Kazakhstan
Tommaso Trevisani
Central Asian Survey, volume 38, issue 3 (September 2019), pp. 381–399

Chapter 5
Appropriating and contesting 'traditional Islam': Central Asian students at the Russian Islamic University in Tatarstan
Dominik Müller
Central Asian Survey, volume 38, issue 3 (September 2019), pp. 400–416

Chapter 6

Traditionalization as a response to state-induced development in rural Tibetan areas of Qinghai, PRC
Jarmila Ptackova
Central Asian Survey, volume 38, issue 3 (September 2019), pp. 417–431

Contributors

Judith Beyer specializes in political and legal anthropology. She conducts long-term ethnographic fieldwork in Central Asia (Kyrgyzstan) and Southeast Asia (Myanmar) and increasingly in Europe. Her research focuses on the anthropology of law, the anthropology of the state, and theories of sociality and social order. Her current thematic interests are the concept of community, common sense, statelessness, existential anthropology, and ethnomethodology. She is the author of *The force of custom. Law and the ordering of everyday life in Kyrgyzstan* (2016) and co-editor of *Ethnographies of the state in Central Asia. Performing politics* (together with Madeleine Reeves and Johan Rasanayagam; 2014). Her second monograph problematizes the category of 'community,' drawing on case studies among Muslims and Hindus in urban Myanmar.

Juliette Cleuziou is an Assistant Professor at the University Lumières-Lyon 2/LADEC, France. She has been working on issues of kinship, gender relations, and marriage economy in Tajikistan, and she is currently leading a two-year programme on death in migration in the post-Soviet Central Asian-Russian space.

Peter Finke specializes in economic anthropology, political economy, and post-socialist transformations. He has worked on pastoral nomadism, identity, cognitive anthropology, and norms and ideologies in Mongolia and Central Asia, where he carried out extensive field research. He is the author of two books: *Variations on Uzbek Identity: Strategic Choices, Cognitive Schemas and Political Constraints in Identification Processes* (2014) and *Nomaden im Transformationsprozess. Kasachen in der post-sozialistischen Mongolei* (2004).

Aijarkyn Kojobekova is an Evaluation and Research Expert of Social Terrain – Unum ltd. United Kingdom – Kyrgyzstan. She holds a PhD in Philosophy. Her research interests are connected with political culture, social memory, and nation building process in Central Asia as well as migration in Eurasia. Currently, she is a focal point of the International Network for the Silk Road Online Platform of UNESCO.

Diana T. Kudaibergenova is the COMPASS Research Associate at the Centre of Development Studies at the University of Cambridge, UK. She studies different intersections of power relations through realms of political sociology dealing with concepts of state, nationalizing regimes, and ideologies. Currently, she is completing her third book manuscript on power, state, and resistance in contemporary art of post-Soviet Eurasia and works on a new project dealing with empowerment.

Dominik Müller studied anthropology, Islamic studies, and political science at the University of Basel and the University of Zurich, Switzerland. He was a visiting researcher at the European Institute of Bilgi University, Istanbul, Turkey, and a project assistant at the Department of Social Work of the Zurich University of Applied Sciences, Switzerland. Since 2013, he has been researching and teaching at the University of Zurich, Switzerland, in the fields of economic anthropology, migration, and transnationalism as well as religious anthropology.

Jarmila Ptackova, PhD, works at the Oriental Institute of the Czech Academy of Sciences, Prague, Czech Republic. She specializes in the study of modern Tibetan society. Her research also focuses on a study of adaptation strategies and adaptation ability of China's minority population to transformed and modernized social and economic environment.

Tommaso Trevisani is an Associate Professor in the Department of Asian, African and Mediterranean Studies at the University of Naples, 'L'Orientale', Italy, where he teaches Societies and Cultures of Central Asia. He researches on agrarian and environmental change; class and industrial work; ritual, marriage, family, and society; state- and nation-building in socialist and post-socialist Central Asia.

INTRODUCTION

Practices of traditionalization in Central Asia

Judith Beyer and Peter Finke

Over the last two centuries, 'tradition'[1] has been invoked in Central Asia by Russian and Soviet regimes, as well as by local Central Asian elites, largely in two ways: either as a deficiency to be overcome (often in juxtaposition to an aspirational 'modernity') or as a quality to be embraced (often in alignment with nationalism). The two are not mutually exclusive or even strictly separate, but the distinction serves well to outline general themes and dynamics in the work of tradition. It is likewise difficult to make clear distinctions between academic analyses and everyday invocations of the term, as they play off one another, and entirely new genres of writing and practice are still emerging. The centrality of tradition in today's Central Asia cannot, however, be denied.

In the first modality – juxtaposition to 'modernity' – large-scale social reforms were introduced and justified by Soviet authorities, who understood themselves to be modern, and set in opposition to 'tradition', which was to be eradicated. Central Asian families were regarded as carriers of 'feudal-patriarchal' ideology (Massell 1975), traditional legal institutions were portrayed as 'backward' (Martin 2001), and 'bride abduction', which still occurs in the region, became an emblem of the 'primitive' (Werner 2009). In all these cases, tradition was framed as the conceptual enemy that needed to be fought and ultimately overcome.

However, alignment with nationalism was never far away even during Soviet times, when various modernization projects were conducted throughout Central Asia in the context of socialist statehood. While socialist statehood was in itself a modern project that had to be constantly negotiated (Kassymbekova 2017), tradition acquired multiple new meanings, just as the concept of 'modernity', as its polar opposite (Eisenstadt 2000), did. Tradition, therefore, became less easy to dismiss by way of (often transparent) juxtaposition to modernity; instead, state officials began aligning tradition with their nation-building initiatives, especially after independence in 1991. In this second modality of alignment, practices of traditionalization allowed new forms of instrumental meaning-making to emerge, thereby providing a foundation upon which the elite could promote tradition as a marker of identity and political reconstruction.

But tradition has never been the exclusive domain of those in power; it has always also been a demotic vehicle for challenge and criticism.[2] The last decade has seen a diversification of what can 'get done' and what is being framed in the name of tradition. Taking into account the scholarly literature that criticizes the very concept of 'invented traditions', the aim of this special issue is to shift attention to understanding traditionalization as a bottom-up process in which elites do not necessarily dictate the course of events, let alone the outcomes.

The concept of tradition in Central Asia

In contemporary Central Asia, the development of tradition as an analytical concept has gone hand in hand with the concept of capitalist modernity, just as it served a socialist cause in the preceding decades. Tradition was introduced and promoted from 'above' by authorities in the newly independent nation-states, who drew on allegedly 'authentic' traditions to claim continuity with a distant past, which allowed them to establish national(ist) narratives that helped legitimize their claims over a certain territory. As 'invented traditions' (Hobsbawm and Ranger 1983), these often newly installed practices, institutions and discourses drew on the concept of tradition to unite a heterogeneous population under one flag. In studying these developments of the last 30 years, scholars have devoted particular attention to elites and intellectuals whose role it had been to codify the kind of tradition that should from now on represent and embody the nation.

By now, we have not only numerous academic publications on these dynamics (e.g. Roy 2000; Tabyshalieva 2000; Hirsch 2005; Morozova 2005; Bergne 2006; Munkh-Erdene 2008; Adams 2010), but also a large number of books and articles written by Central Asian elites themselves. Intellectuals have engaged in what Hutchinson (1987, 1999) has called 'cultural nationalism' in order to increase social legitimacy. 'Writing tradition' is by now an established literary genre that the presidents of all five post-Soviet Central Asian republics have engaged in: Turkmenistan's *Rukhnama* (Nyazov 2005) and *Adamnama* (Berdymukhammedov 2013); Kazakhstan's *Epicenter of Peace* and *The Kazakhstan Way* (Nazarbaev 2001, 2008); Kyrgyzstan's *Kyrgyz Statehood and the Popular Epic 'Manas'* (Akaev 2003);[3] Uzbekistan's *High Morality: An Invincible Force* (Karimov 2008; see also Kendzior 2014); and Tajikistan's *The Tajiks in the Mirror of History: From the Aryans to the Samanids* (Rahmon 2009).

Although newly independent nation-states might 'set out to purify traditions of foreign influences' (Noyes 2009, 242), the propagation of nationalist tradition continues to be significantly supported from the 'outside' as well. International organizations and foreign experts align their new programmes and projects with the countries' 'rich historical pasts', and local NGOs often go along with these notions and the quickly established idiom of tradition to secure financial support or attract foreign supporters. Examples include tourist initiatives that advertise 'nomadic ways of life' and 'community-based' approaches to issues ranging from disaster management to volunteerism, development in the more general sense, and alternative dispute resolution that encourages working with local organizations. The globally recognized rhetoric of 'cultural heritage' and 'indigenous rights' is also being increasingly invoked in Central Asian discourses, where it organizes the heterogeneity (Eriksen 2007, 10) of different ethnic groups or corporate interests.[4]

Although Eric Hobsbawm and Terence Ranger (1983), who first coined the term 'invented tradition' in the context of postcolonial deconstruction, do not essentialize tradition, they have been criticized for 'draw[ing] a distinction between unself-conscious custom perpetuated by natural communities, such as villages, and self-conscious traditions invented by unnatural ones, namely nations and states' (Jolly 1992, 51). And while Marshall Sahlins (1999, 399) rejects the concept as an 'easy functionalist dismissal of the people's claims of cultural distinction', Michael Herzfeld reminds us that '*all* culture is in this sense invented' (2014, 214, emphasis in the original) and urges us to look at how and in what contexts concepts are put to use. This is what, according to Ranger (1993, 63), the two authors had in mind when they were investigating 'a specific historical period, in which ... traditions were peculiarly frequently invented rather than customs continuing to evolve'.

Briggs (1996, 463) has further criticized literature on the 'invention of tradition' for 'extend[ing] and legitimat[ing] scholarly control over the discourses of Others'. He emphasizes the need not only to understand the context in which discursive authority – that is, authority over the interpretation of tradition – is constructed, but also to acknowledge that what has often been characterized as fictitious has become part of the lived experience of the people with whom we work. How do actors make claims to represent cultural constructions, and which of these claims become successful and which do not? John and Jean Comaroff demonstrated in *Ethnicity, Inc.* (2009) that there is no reason to believe that the business of 'inventing tradition' would come to a halt in the post-colonial era. On the contrary, in the post-colonial era,

> The recuperation of 'tradition' under the impact of Ethnicity, Inc. may have the effect of reifying 'culture' as a thing in and of itself. And, in the upshot, its products and practices, rendered as intellectual property, may be more or less directed at the market. But, invariably, the process also has an impact on everyday conduct: on those less-objectified, unremarked upon ways of doing things. (75)

It is on this latter aspect, that is, the impact of tradition on everyday life, that our attention lies in this special issue. We want to move beyond probing the 'authenticity' of particular 'traditional practices'. Rather than deconstructing tradition in order to do away with it, we see here a site of necessary engagement. Tradition does matter in Central Asia, as it does in Africa and in Europe: it aggregates people, motivates individual and collective action, informs policy, public debates, law, and representation, and is – despite its often enough strategic inception – affectively powerful. Thus, to investigate the processes of traditionalization is not just an act of 'Othering', as Briggs claims, but also an effort to investigate and understand phenomena that are very real in the lives of the people we observe. And like any other aspect of society, these processes entail elements of invention that – once brought into existence – take on a life of their own and become highly relevant. Hence, putting aside possible structural differences between the inventions of demotic actors and those of elites, we focus instead on the practical ways in which tradition is put to use, by whom and to what ends. Often, the elites' projects of traditionalization and those of ordinary actors speak to and rely on each other in a rather dialectical way. While a great deal of discussion has centred on what tradition entails and what it does not, including the question of invention and ownership, less attention has been devoted to investigating how tradition is enacted, enforced or motivated – in short, how it is 'done'. When does tradition emerge as a line of argumentation, and how is it (materially) manifested? We also ask where and around what issues invocations of and discussions about tradition arise. Continuing to highlight the importance of tradition in ongoing nation-building processes, this special issue therefore focuses attention on the 'everydayification' (to translate quite literally Weber's *Veralltäglichung*) of tradition in arenas ranging from political demonstrations (Beyer and Kojobekova) and industrial workers' gatherings (Trevisani) to institutions of religious education (Müller), minority communities (Ptackova), wedding celebrations (Cleuziou) and the Internet (Kudaibergenova).

The empirical data provided in all of the contributions suggest that there is in each site at the very least a stable working definition of what tradition is, and – as stated above – the debates over its extent and its qualities are an inevitable part of the phenomenon. In this set of texts, we work with context-sensitive translations only and question our own assumptions about the characteristics the concept of tradition might entail, remembering that while 'traditional practices' might be presented as age-old, long-established and often uncodified principles, they are also deeply embodied, gendered, age-specific and all-encompassing ways of conduct. According to Mould (2005, 268), we can speak of traditionalization when a practice is communally recognized as traditional. Cleuziou (this issue) shows how, in the name of *an'ana*, wedding festivities in Tajikistan constitute events where participants construct 'the traditional'. In doing so, new practices and goods can become integrated into this domain as they are debated over and receive approval or, in some cases, are simply accepted without being questioned or challenged.

Tradition, in the words of Glassie (1995, 395), 'spreads into association with adjacent, related, equally indispensable terms'. This finding is in line with how, for example, the entry for the Kyrgyz term *salt* in the Kyrgyz ethnographic dictionary is composed: it specifies the term by referring to other terms with similar meanings. In this case *ürp-adat*, *nark*, *yrym-zhyrym*, and *kaada-salt* are given as explanations or definitions (Karataev and Eraliev 2005, 402–403). Beyer (2016, 6) has argued that in Kyrgyzstan, the word *salt* itself can be used interchangeably with *adat* (usually translated as customary law), as well as with all of the aforementioned terms, even though references to *salt* are much more common.[5] As the concept of *salt*, like the other concepts that the authors of this special issue explore, is intentionally ambiguous in both scholarly and emic discourses, efforts to delineate and translate these notions fail when taken out of context.

Tradition as practice and as institution

In this special issue, we are taking a praxeological approach to tradition that emphasizes how actors strategically demonstrate, imitate, claim and negotiate tradition. Understood in such a way, tradition remains always fragmentary, 'a fluid and transforming agent with no real end' (Hunn 1993, 13). Of course, tradition is not an agent, though it may be presented as such by its practitioners or other stakeholders. Methodologically, it is important to focus on and differentiate between what actors do, what they say they do, and what they say they should do in the name of tradition. Actors are not 'cultural dupes' (Garfinkel 1967); they are reflective and aware of their own and others' behaviour. They reason about their everyday lives just as anthropologists reason about them carrying out their everyday lives. Coming from this angle, practices of traditionalization can be fruitfully understood as exercises in sense-making by the actors themselves – to themselves and to one another (see also Mould 2005). From an analytical perspective, we treat traditionalization as the institutionalization of social practice, informed by – and, in turn, informing – cultural models.[6]

The early socialist regime explicitly aimed to destroy traditions that were believed to legitimize inequalities in Central Asia and were, therefore, considered harmful to societal development. Today, in contrast, international organizations and NGOs often tend to rely on so-called traditional leaders and hierarchies to implement development projects, thus sometimes reinforcing local inequalities in the name of stability and general well-being (Heathershaw 2009). The degree to which these endeavours were successful can be studied by examining comparatively how a 'traditional' nomadic way of life is perceived today in such places as Kazakhstan, Kyrgyzstan and Mongolia. In all three, picturesque images of yurts and mounted shepherds abound, but in Kazakhstan at least it continues to be seen as a backwards and, by and large, embarrassing lifestyle, no matter how traditional it may be, while in Mongolia it is still a vibrant part of the public imagination and an important point of reference and pride (Finke 2004; Vuillemenot 2009).

We should regard tradition not as an object of fixed history but as part of a process of identity formation. The concept is thus analytically freed from being treated as a paradoxical object of iron-clad history that endures or – in a movement of revitalization – is reintroduced into our present time.[7] As a particular type of practice that always needs to be explored in its concrete institutional and interactional context at a particular time, tradition can only be judged from the present. It is an interpretative concept, not a descriptive one. Tradition therefore reflects the tensions between continuity and change, or predictability and flexibility. In rapidly transforming societies, however, it can be expected that there will be more variation in the interpretation and acceptance (or disavowal) of tradition. This gives ample opportunities for cultural entrepreneurs to come up with their own readings. New wedding ceremonies, the role of lineage or village elders, the necessity of religious piety or female purity are all cases in point that serve – or are intended to serve – the interests of those actors pursuing them. On a discursive level, this is portrayed as a dichotomy between modernizers and conservatives, but in everyday life there are many more facets to be found between the two ends of the spectrum. On a political level, many cases of retraditionalization can be interpreted as paths by which powerful local and national actors try to redefine social order in their own interests and impose a corresponding set of rules of the game on everyone around. We thus need to pay attention to those actors who have the means to define a situation (Bailey 1969).

Being the result of ongoing negotiation processes among different groups of actors, tradition is fluid and always prone to change. At the same time, to be meaningful, practices of traditionalization need a certain degree of durability and predictability. Otherwise, as institutional arrangements, they would lose credibility both in ideological terms and as guidelines for mutually expected patterns of acting (Ensminger 1992). Empirically speaking, there is, moreover, a wide range of rule adherence. Some traditions exist merely 'on paper' and have very little relevance in daily life (such as national dances or outfits worn only on specific occasions that may or may not have been more widespread in the past). Others seem more deeply ingrained – such as strong sanctions on inappropriate behaviour towards women or elderly people – and disregarding them may lead to serious contestations and eventually coercive acts of rectification. Even if the sanctions imposed are informal, they may cause severe stress and social exclusion.[8]

When and how does tradition change? One simple yet insightful economic answer to this is when relative prices and the corresponding bargaining power of different actors change (Ensminger 1992; Knight 1992). There is some merit to this idea. In the early

1990s, when most of Central Asia went through deep crises and people saw their livelihoods deteriorating overnight, wedding expenses posed a great challenge to household budgets. Different strategies to cope with this have been identified, and all reflect back on understandings of tradition. Among Kazakhs in Mongolia, as well as in other parts of the region, one way to restrict the size and expense of wedding ceremonies was to switch to a ritualized form of bride abduction: everyone knew in advance what would happen, but still the family of the girl would not participate in the event itself, cutting attendance (and costs) in half (Finke 2004). With the economic recovery in more recent years, weddings have become – as they have in all parts of Central Asia – an important tool to demonstrate a family's social standing and are celebrated as lavishly as possible. Today, the ceremony is announced months in advance, and the preparations for horse races and wrestling competitions leave no space for abductions. In Kyrgyzstan, we have a different situation: even though bride abduction has been punishable since pre-Soviet times, with the maximum prison sentence being increased in the Criminal Code in 2013, and despite intensive lobbying against the practice by local and international NGOs, bride abduction persists.[9] In Tajikistan, in contrast, ceremonies are rarely announced far in advance because they greatly depend on men returning from their labour migration to Russia, which is often difficult to foresee, and on the remittances they bring along (see Cleuziou, this issue).

Appeals to tradition can serve to disguise the unequal distributional effects of specific rules within a population. The marriage patterns just described are a case in point: the trend towards ever more ostentatious ceremonies and displays of wealth, as in parts of Kazakstan, apparently began as a competition among the leading families within the communities. In their efforts to outperform one another, new arenas and opportunities emerged to demonstrate wealth and status. These conspicuous displays of tradition eventually encouraged others – including the less well-off – to try to keep up with the elites, which for many intensified debt and financial precarity.[10] Another illustrative case of power asymmetries disguised by contemporary practices of traditionalization is the re-emergence of patronage networks, camouflaged as extended kin relations that serve all sides and, like bride abduction, are described as an inextricable part of traditional culture (Ismailbekova 2017). This camouflage of factual hierarchies as performances of egalitarian ideals indicates that tradition in Central Asia can cover up or legitimize existing inequalities. Powerful actors may use traditional concepts, or sometimes invent them, to serve their own purposes or to justify how institutional rules distribute costs and benefits, as in the case of patronage networks. That is to say, recourse to tradition in support networks might secure or even increase one's (superior) position in society.

Tradition as cultural model

We hold that there is no single authoritative point of view from which to decide what should be considered tradition in any particular setting. In consequence, there is no monopoly on tradition, despite the strong naturalistic and unitary conception of the term that many actors employ. At the same time, there are limits to the range of interpretations and instrumentalizations of tradition that have to do with prevailing local cultural models of how things are supposed to be done as well as power hierarchies that determine which actors can – with authority – determine what should count as traditional. This is not to say that people do not act habitually, but to identify such enactment of cultural models as 'tradition' is an active intervention, a purposeful framing, that has real consequences.

To refer to cultural models or schemes acknowledges that it is possible and productive to abstract certain shared understandings about how things in the world are connected to observed behaviour. But such cultural models are always unevenly distributed in a population, and we can never quite prove that any such a model guided a decision (whether consciously or unconsciously). Going back to the early criticism of Hobsbawm and Ranger (see above), we do not espouse a strict distinction between 'unself-conscious custom ... and self-conscious traditions'. Rather, we proceed empirically: some models are more easily articulated, others less so; in any case, we assume that actors are in principle capable of the reflexivity needed to both identify and proclaim such models. Cultural models with not only a practical but also a moral component, such as respect for elders, are especially conducive to effective public articulation. When invoking cultural models, people make statements about how things ought to be done properly, and how broad the range of acceptable behaviour is in a given context. They also find their expressions in proverbs, morality tales and the wisdom of the elders, central elements of what counts as tradition. Some cultural models may leave little room for flexibility and alternatives, such as those related to religion or gender relations; others may be less strict. Such ideas about 'traditional' and 'proper' ways of life (often used interchangeably) are ideological in that they explain the world in terms of rightful hierarchies – or challenge them.

Cultural models of tradition are transmitted from generation to generation by way of domestic socialization and public policies. They can also, however, lose currency. Insights from cognitive anthropology show that those ideas transmitted in early childhood have an especially strong and lasting impact on people's understanding of the world. Cultural models, then, enable people to more easily share understandings of tradition, which still can be shaped by individual experience; they are both durable and fluid in the course of one's lifetime, as Strauss and Quinn (1997) put it. Many of these models are only partially conscious and are thus hard to access. While there is debate on how to define the respective units of reference and the number of adherents necessary to call any model a cultural one, many of those schemas that make up tradition are internalized to such a degree that they seem to be the obvious and often the only possible way of doing things. This is enhanced by the terminology that declares something to be a tradition, endowing it with an aura of authenticity, eternalness and even sacredness. One example of this is the celebrations for Nowruz all across Central Asia.[11] Other practices are obviously new, but may nevertheless quickly gain recognition, such as the independence day in each of the new Central Asian states.

Cultural models that concern social relations have a tendency to develop into stereotypes (Brubaker, Loveman, and Stamatov 2004). For the case of tradition, this means that people may well understand the biases and asymmetries in unequal treatment that they promote (for example, gender- or age-based differences) but be less aware of the underlying cultural basis. Cognition studies offer the related insight that different schemes or models are connected with one another in ways that are likewise difficult to penetrate consciously. For example, the perceived lack of 'modernity' among minorities in China, as described by Ptackova in this issue, is part of an emically ordered ethnic (or even 'racial') hierarchy that is particularly difficult to overcome, in part because it is shared to a certain degree even by the people negatively affected by this very taxonomy.

Its basis in shared knowledge (which we are calling 'models' here) also puts certain limits on the flexibility of tradition and, hence, its susceptibility to manipulation. A new model has to make sense to actors: the further away from established ideas it is, the more effort has to be spent to implement it (and the greater the risk of failure; see Wagner 1975). This is to say that the invention or transformation of tradition is often more gradual than abrupt, incremental rather than radical. A radical shift in existing models, such as if someone suddenly tried to proclaim that Kyrgyz had from time immemorial been sedentary agriculturalists rather than free-ranging herders, would demand the investment of significant resources, financial as well as rhetorical. Even not entirely implausible claims, such as that promoted by some intellectuals in the early 1990s, that shamanism had been the original religion of Kazaks and should be restored as such, have been largely futile because they could not be reconciled with the way people conceive of themselves (and possibly for other reasons as well).[12] It may, therefore, not always be possible to predict how tradition will change or which efforts towards its invention or reinstallation will succeed.

Nevertheless, when it comes to practice, tradition occasions a permanent struggle over meaning and requires constant renegotiation, as is amply demonstrated by the contributions in this special issue. This is partly because tradition is inherently ambivalent and fuzzy – more so than its promoters would like it to be. Some purportedly well-established Central Asian practices, such as child betrothal and the levirate, are in fact rejected by a significant portion of the population; others are disliked but still accepted as a matter of fact. An interesting case is the attitude towards alcohol in most of Muslim Central Asia. Pretty much everyone is aware that drinking alcohol violates religious prescriptions, yet consumption patterns have remained consistently high and are linked to the performance of traditional events such as weddings, circumcision ceremonies and national holidays. Many such ambivalent practices are now often labelled as a type of tradition – as 'our way of doing things' – even if they understand them as relatively recent innovations (Zanca 2003; Finke 2014).[13]

Beyer (2016) has demonstrated that designating practices as traditional is one way people can react to social change; tradition is thus never in the past, but always in the present (see also Eisenstadt 1973). Jolly (1992, 63), in a similar vein, suggests that scholars ought to 'look more carefully and comparatively at the encoding of past–present relations in the variety of symbolic constitutions of tradition' instead of trying to identify 'real pasts' in contrast to lay people's inventions of it. Towards a more granular analysis, Mould (2005, 257) reminds us that we can differentiate 'conscious and explicit efforts of traditionalization from inherent or implicit factors that feed or reinforce a tradition'. 'The past' is, moreover, no longer the key resource, as Hobsbawm and Ranger had it, but only one option among many for how to tell stories about oneself and about others.

To summarize, practices of traditionalization can thus be both inclusive and exclusive, integrative as well as divisive (Cocq 2014). While elites might impose their views and interests and try to force others to accept them as the (new) rules of the game, demotic actors can always reinterpret and challenge top-down models to a certain degree. Investigating tradition as practice allows one to study not only how tradition comes into being in the first place and is legitimized, but also how it is challenged and refuted. Though it draws its rhetorical appeal from its seemingly stable and non-negotiable character, tradition should be understood as always contestable and fragmentary. Actors can only ever achieve common ground on what the notion should entail in concrete situations.

Approaching tradition from these theoretical angles, we concentrate on exploring three dominant themes in the contributions to this special issue that allow productive cross-referencing: gender, authority and religion.

Fields of traditionalization

Doing gender

While tradition has been encouraged and put to use by the various governmental elites in Central Asia for the purpose of nation-building, it has regularly been discouraged by those same actors once women's rights and their representation come into play.[14] Women's issues have always been linked to tradition, as it is very often through discourses on and practices related to gender that tradition can manifest itself visibly and publicly. This is particularly the case when the matter concerns religion and family (Akiner 1997; Werner 2009; Kocaoglu 2009). After the forced unveiling campaign (*hujum*) in 1927 (Northrop 2004), which took place mostly in Tajikistan and Uzbekistan but is well known throughout Central Asia, women were forced to participate in the Soviet workforce while still fulfilling all of the expectations of their roles as wives, mothers and daughters (-in-law) (Tett 1994; Dragadze 1994).

State nationalisms and movements of national liberation are very often intrinsically linked to conceptions of gender hierarchy (Yuval-Davis 1997), and this observation holds throughout Central Asia as well: 'In the context of post-Soviet Central Asian nationalisms, the elaboration of national unity, authenticity, and identity inscribes itself in the idea of "returning to tradition", in order to mark – to varying degrees in each state – distance or rupture with the Soviet promotion of the "women's question"' (Cleuziou and Direnberger 2016, 196). State measures as much as nationalist groups tend to restrict women's mobility, their control over their own bodies, and their political participation through various policies and actions (regarding, for example, social provisioning, clothing, marriage, etc.), and try to circumscribe their sphere of activity to the frame of the household. In this context, gender activism and equality may be dismissed as incompatible with traditional gender norms (Cleuziou and Direnberger 2016, 198).

Tabyshalieva (2000, 55) has argued that, after independence, Central Asian women were 'caught up in three rings of discrimination, influenced by traditions of patriarchy, Soviet ideals, and images from the West'. Patriarchal traditions, for her, include the demands to marry early, give birth to many children (particularly sons) and still bear sole responsibility for the household. After the collapse of the Soviet Union, the latter burden has become even heavier, as social security provisions are no longer in place. Bride abduction has become more frequent in Kyrgyzstan in the last two decades. As for polygamy, it is illegal according to state laws, but nevertheless continues to be practised in Kyrgyzstan. In the context of changing gender ideologies, new publications have stressed 'gender neotraditionalism' (Megoran 1999; Johnson and Robinson 2006, 2009). Commercio (2015, 529–30) argues that 'retraditionalization resonates with young, urban, educated women', thus, those who are 'least likely … to embrace traditional values'. She has addressed the concept of retraditionalization in regard to her topic of interest – women approaching adulthood – from a perspective that is similar to ours in this special issue, namely, as an empirically oriented inquiry. She found that university-educated women in both Kyrgyzstan and Tajikistan sympathize with traditional gender roles.

In Kyrgyzstan, in the context of another constitutional reform (for background, see Beyer 2015), so-called 'higher values' (Russ.: *norma o vysshikh tsennostiakh*) such as 'respect for the elderly' and 'love of the Motherland' have been added to the preamble of the constitution. Along with these suggestions comes a respecification of the term 'family' from 'a union of two people' to the gender-specific 'a union between a man and a woman'.[15] Thus while in practical everyday life this union is increasingly frequently fractured due to labour migration, polygamy and high divorce rates, the law emphasizes a traditional image of the family, as if wanting to counter *de facto* developments on the ground. In this special issue, we investigate how women deal with this predicament and how they try to bend practices of traditionalization to their own advantage.

The power of authority

In this special issue, we understand authority not as the exercise of individual will or as an office (cf. Weber 1922; for Central Asia, see Jones Luong 2002, 68), but as the effect of a co-emergent practice of legitimization: we speak of authority when respect is accorded to the holders of particular types of skills or knowledge (or direct access to the divine), who in turn display what others regard as appropriate behaviour (Beyer 2016). Since authority is relational and derives from how people interact with others (Blumer 1969, 7), it should be seen as a basic aspect of human interactional behaviour rather than an individual capacity in itself (Peabody 1968). Authority is always dependent on the acknowledgement others are willing to show (Abu-Lughod 1986, 103; Arendt 1986); nevertheless, authority and power have commonalities, such as a hierarchical component and their relationality (Arendt 1993, 93; Wolf 1999).

Since the advent of poststructuralism and Foucault's work on power, however, authority seems to have received less attention. Foucault's (1979, 93) famous statement that we can find power 'everywhere' might have influenced researchers to explore hierarchical relationships predominantly in terms of power rather than authority. But Foucault was less interested in concrete interactions, and more in discursive formations. Those espousing interactionalist approaches are predominantly concerned with situated struggles, which makes them reluctant to offer their analyses in terms of power.[16] Building on a contemporary social science literature that has increasingly emphasized the consensual or collusive aspects of power in addition to its coercive nature (Lukes 1986, 2005), the case studies presented here suggest that while tradition can be realized through institutionalized power, new organizations need to be staffed with people who are respected and can express their opinion in the name of tradition. These actors can then frame new practices and behaviour as traditional. In general terms, focusing on the interplay of power and authority offers us a more sophisticated understanding of how stratified relationships between actors are emerging in the context of traditionalization. The invocation of tradition can then be understood as an authenticating strategy: the traditional becomes a resource actively manipulated for specific and often personal ends (Appadurai 1995). Thus, it is to tradition that people attribute the power to render a practice, an idea, a place or an object authentic.

In addition to this analytical consideration, throughout Central Asia there is also an emic distinction between the concepts of power and authority. Power is attributed primarily to the (Soviet) state and to those individuals who are seen to be connected to it, which is why the Russian word *vlast'* (power) is often used even in Central Asian languages. Authority, on the other hand, refers to a culturally established pattern of behaviour entailing clearly demarcated roles that need to be performed and acted out in front of others if one's behaviour and actions are to be recognized as worthy of authority. This has consequences particularly for women who, in the context of having lost their husbands to wars in Soviet times, high divorce rates, labour migration of men to Russia, and the emerging debates on legalizing polygamy (as are currently taking place in Kyrgyzstan, Tajikistan and Kazakhstan[17]), have had to and continue to fulfil roles traditionally attributed to men only, for example that of being the head of a household (Ismailbekova 2016; Cleuziou, this issue).

The intertwining of religion and tradition

The third field of tradition we want to examine in greater detail is the manifestations of and local negotiations regarding religion. In one of his decrees, then president of Kyrgyzstan Almazbek Atambaev observed 'the weakening of traditional Islam', noting that 'contradictions in the Muslim community led to a loosening of the traditional Hanafi Sunni Islam'.[18] In the name of 'the defence of national culture and national identity', a 'fundamental revision of the principles and methods of the interaction between state and religion' have been put in place since then. While Atambaev's proclamations contradict the academic discourse of the 1990s, which asserted that an 'Islamic revival' was taking place in the region (Collins 2007; McGlinchey 2009), they are in line with Pelkmans's (2017) more recent argument that traditional versions of Islam (and Christianity) held rather limited appeal for those who developed an interest in practising religion in Kyrgyzstan. Some turned to new religious movements instead, such as Christian Pentecostalism and the Muslim Tablighi Jamaat. Nowadays, however, according to Commercio (2015), traditional religious and family values are accepted throughout both Kyrgyzstan and Tajikistan. In the latter context, reformist movements of Islam have been active since the late 1960s (Dudoignon and Noack 2014).

Beyer (2006, 2016) suggests that the contradictory findings among scholars mirror local debates over the interpretation of practices and institutions as either traditional, religious, or both, and that it was precisely the overlap between cultural and religious repertoires that allowed actors to act more freely (see also Rasanayagam 2011, 2014). When Jones (2017), in her recent edited volume on Islam in Central Asia, advocates discarding the term 'revival' and speaks of 'transformation' instead, she acknowledges these 'competing discourses', which are by no means limited to Central Asia.[19] Such a change of wording, however, would hardly meet the approval of many people in the region, who – for better or for worse – do experience the recent changes as a form of re-emergence and a regaining of importance on the part of religion in general.

Introducing the case studies

This set of articles offers new insights into the shared theme of traditionalization. Their theoretical reflections and ethnographic case studies promise relevance beyond the field of Central Asian studies. The articles are based on papers given at the 2015 conference of the European Society for Central Asian Studies, titled 'Central Asia in the XXI Century: Historical Trajectories, Contemporary Challenges and Everyday Encounters', and held at the University of Zurich. The authors represented in this special issue met for a second time at the University of Konstanz in November 2017 to discuss draft versions of their articles and work on the common theme. We have thus accumulated a rich and well-matched palette of ethnographic case studies that approach traditionalization from different angles while retaining a common focus on the various practical realizations of tradition.

In 'Women of Protest, Men of Applause', Judith Beyer and Aijarkyn Kojobekova explore two unexpected kinds of strongly gendered activists and the ways they tap into practices of traditionalization in the context of Kyrgyzstan's recent turbulent political past. The different degrees of acceptance these actors have found is grounded in the respective standing and traditional stereotypes of men and women.

In 'Traditionalization, or the Making of Reputation', Juliette Cleuziou explores the performances of widows during their daughters' weddings, as they shoulder the double burden of performing as both mother and father to comply with expected traditional behaviour. Even if success – measured by the duration of marriages – is uncertain, given the high rates of divorce in the country, these widows strive to protect their daughters from the bad reputation of being fatherless.

Further exploring the theme of gender, Diana Kudaibergenova addresses the impact social media in Kazakhstan and Russia can have on local actors. Her article, 'The Body Globalized and Retraditionalized', shows how people using platforms such as Instagram for their own personal liberation expose themselves to global discourses on gender, body and sex, while others tap into public discussions and personal online profiles to circulate and strengthen discourses of traditionalization beyond the private, local and national spheres. All three articles focus on the complex emotion of shame (*uiat*; also 'shame-anxiety') that actors invoke to justify, rationalize or stigmatize their own or others' behaviour.

Probing the question of what happens to tradition once it is dislocated from its seemingly proper domain, Tommaso Trevisani's article 'The Veterans' Gala' investigates how, in a steel company in Karaganda, in southern Kazakhstan, a council of elders is being created by the company's manager to keep the growing dissatisfaction among employees at bay. Here, traditionalization recurs as a practice that both affirms and challenges industrial leadership in labour conflicts.

Dominik Müller writes on negotiating 'traditional Islam' among Central Asian students at the Russian Islamic University in Kazan, Tatarstan. He argues that for these youths, studying Islam as it is currently promoted by the Russian government is often a coping mechanism to deal with economic uncertainty while their parents hope to secure their children's moral upbringing. Besides being an expression of religious piety, it is thus also a way of increasing one's future job opportunities by combining Islamic topics with secular programmes such as law or economics.

Jarmila Ptackova, in 'Traditionalization as a Response to State-induced Development in Rural Tibetan Areas of Qinghai, PRC', investigates the impact of Chinese modernization schemes in minority areas. For several decades, the expansion of infrastructure and economic restructuring to the western provinces has been a dominant theme in the literature and has often been interpreted as an attempt to assimilate the minority populations to the Han Chinese way of life. Questioning the allegedly solely negative impacts of these developments on the lives of Tibetans (who in fact often welcome modernization efforts), Ptackova goes on to explore responses that include a retreat from and a reappraisal of indigenous tradition. Examples of this are language use, food, handicrafts and rituals, as well as their adaptations in movies and the tourism sector.

The future of tradition

Practices of traditionalization can be understood as efforts to link the present to the past, thereby emphasizing a continuity of practices, material culture, and institutions that in turn furthers claims to authenticity and historical or even mythical continuity. These claims have been appropriated by Central Asian states in their efforts to develop particular national identity projects – but they have also always been part and parcel of ordinary people's cultural strategies. As tradition continues to matter in contemporary times, this special issue explores new arenas of its application, with a focus on the general population more than on elite actors. Without a doubt, tradition provides political actors and local elites with a source of legitimacy for an existing social order or for an intended direction of change. As such, tradition is commonly a 'weapon of the strong', to invert Scott's (1987) famous phrase. It is of particular importance – if the respective recourse is to be accepted and successful – to create an aura of seemingly indisputable facts, such as the right of elderly men, but not of women, to engage in local power games. However, comparatively few traditions and discourses are beyond contestation, and in the post-socialist period many regions, especially Central Asia but elsewhere as well, have seen the rise and fall of efforts to (re-)establish allegedly age-old habits and customs.

In this special issue we therefore set out to answer the following questions: Who needs tradition, and what is it being put to use for? How can authority emerge from referencing tradition? And who can control, police and oversee its associated practices? The various case studies illustrate not only its strategic use in diverse settings across Central Asia, but also its unintended side effects. Moreover, we analyse current developments in the region from an interactional angle that has thus far been little tested on material from Central Asia; this offers insights that allow comparison to processes of traditionalization reported throughout the world.

We argue that inequality and power asymmetries are constant features of traditionalization processes. Central Asia is no exception. After decades of socialist rule, with its own traditional practices and ideologies, the search for new fields of meaning and for the resurrection of earlier hierarchies has been successful in some realms and less so in others, as the articles in this special issue demonstrate. As time goes by, new and old traditions become institutionalized yet again, allowing their own dynamics of a seemingly self-explanatory and authoritative nature to unfold. Being enmeshed in broader cultural models of proper attitudes and the structuring of society, those with less power face an uphill battle to promote their own concepts and demands.

In Central Asia, practices of traditionalization are thus closely related to the transformation of the formerly socialist order and the emergence of often highly stratified societies. It would therefore be misleading to simply attribute them to the power of conservative segments of society. Rather, traditionalization is part of a dialectical way of ordering that is negotiated between demotic actors and the various power holders on both the domestic and the national level. It lends actors at the national level an aura of legitimacy, even if the misuses and manipulations seem quite obvious, while allowing those at the local level to manoeuvre, stake alternative claims and display acts of resistance on the ground.

Notes

1. For better readability, we will put the term 'tradition' in quotation marks only when referencing the opinion of others.
2. See Dubuisson (2011, 2017) for the case of *aitys* poetry in Kazakhstan, and Beyer (2016) for the invocation of tradition in the Kyrgyz context.
3. Almazbek Atambaev, the former president of Kyrgyzstan, has not written books any yet, but has already announced that he will do so during his retirement.
4. In recent years there has been increasing reference to (cultural) heritage in the literature on Central Asia (see e.g. McGuire 2017 and, from the perspective of critical heritage studies, Paskaleva 2016, which is an entire special issue bearing the title 'Memory and Commemoration in Central Asia').
5. Likewise, in his definition of *adat*, a concept that is also known throughout Central Asia, Clifford Geertz (2000) draws on German legal anthropologist Franz von Benda-Beckmann's (1979) discussion of the term: 'In his [Benda-Beckmann's] glossary, the word is "defined" as "tradition, custom, law, morality, political system, legal system" which, except for the omission of "etiquette" and "ritual", is about the size of it' (Geertz 2000, 210).
6. We use 'institutions' here according to Douglas North's (1990, 3) definition as 'rules of the game'. This includes a broad spectrum of social regulations, from everyday practices of greeting to multilevel arrangements of property rights and law. Most importantly, institutions entail mutual expectations about how things are supposed to be done, as well as formal or informal sanctions for disregarding such expectations. However, due to the restrictions they impose on possible ways of acting, institutions may always be disputed and are prone to continual change. In fact, according to North, one can only speak of an institution if people follow the rule to the extent necessary to maintain mutual expectations (see also Ensminger 1992; Finke 2004).
7. A. L. Kroeber's (1948) classic anthropological definition of tradition – the 'internal handing on through time' (411) – is still very much in line with the commonsensical understanding.
8. For lack of a better term, we label both of these – the more superficial ones as well as the internalized patterns of behaviour – 'tradition'; together they constitute a continuum along which one and the same act can fall at different points depending on the individual, the situation or the temporal context.
9. In their 2015 report, the UN Committee on the Elimination of Discrimination against Women described bride abduction in Kyrgyzstan as the result of 'discriminatory stereotypes, negative traditional attitudes and harmful practices' (4), and urged authorities 'to address the traditional cultural attitudes and underlying causes of bride kidnapping' (6). This approach demonstrates a clear failure to differentiate between explanans and explanandum.
10. Personal correspondence with Dinara Abildenova.
11. Nowruz, also known as the Persian (or Iranian) New Year, is celebrated on the vernal equinox and marks the end of winter and the beginning of spring.
12. When it comes to traditional medicine, however, Penkala-Gawecka (2013) argues that we are currently witnessing a revival in 'shamanic illness' – the life-altering 'illness' a person must go through to become a shaman – in Kazakhstan, which she attributes to a governmental reappraisal that has established 'folk medicine' as national heritage as well as to newly emerging biomedical discourses.
13. In recent years there have been efforts to prohibit alcohol. Among the Islamist groups, obviously, total abstinence is unconditional, but many more Kazaks and Kyrgyz have replaced

vodka with *qimiz*, or fermented mare's milk, as the national (mildly) alcoholic beverage. It is now increasingly common not to serve vodka during life-cycle ceremonies, or to do so only in secret. People justify this less on religious grounds and more with reference to the traditional role and medicinal values of *qimiz* – which allows even local imams to consume it.

14. Explicitly gender-focused publications have predominantly looked at women's issues. Studies that address manhood, fatherhood, male youth or the construction of male personhood (Reeves 2010; Roche 2014; Schröder 2017; Thibault 2017) often do not approach their topic from a gender perspective, and despite our awareness that migration shapes the construction of manhood in profound ways, we still lack in-depth studies on this topic. However, Kandiyoti (1988, 2007) and Harris (2004) have opened up the debate, and Kamp (2009), Billaud (2015), Cleuziou and Direnberger (2016), as well as Cleuziou, Beyer and Kojobekova, and Kudaibergenova in this special issue are recent examples that address gender as an analytical category rather than a descriptive one.
15. See *Vykhrest* (27 January 2017). "The victims of Russia's ultra-conservatism are the Russian people themselves." Arykbaev (29 August 2016). "Initsiatory dorabotali popravi v konstitutsiyu - chto izmenilos'?" https://kloop.kg/blog/2016/08/29/initsiatory-dorabotali-popravki-v-konstitutsiyu-chto-izmenilos/, accessed 3 June 2019. We can observe similar developments in Russia, where the loosening of laws against domestic violence was justified in the name of 'traditional values' (https://www.opendemocracy.net/od-russia/antonina-vikhrest/victims-of-russia-s-ultra-conservativism-are-russian-people-themselves, accessed 3 June 2019; see also Kudaibergenova, this issue).
16. See Girke (2015) for an example of the negotiation of authority among situated actors that complicates any straightforward understanding of power. In contrast, anthropologists working in a new institutionalist framework tend to focus on issues of power rather than authority (Ensminger 1992; Finke 2004).
17. See the interview with Commercio and Cleuziou at CAAN (Central Asian Analytical Network), 11 May 2016 (http://caa-network.org/archives/7076, accessed 3 June 2019).
18. Presidential Decree 'O realizatsii resheniia Soveta oborony Kyrgyzskoi Respubliki o gosudarstvennoi politike v religioznoi sfere', 7 February 2014.
19. Talal Asad (1983) suggested studying Islam in general as a 'discursive tradition'.

Acknowledgment

The authors thank Juliette Cleuziou and Felix Girke for their helpful comments on this introduction.

Disclosure statement

No potential conflict of interest was reported by the authors.

References

Abu-Lughod, L. 1986. *Veiled Sentiments: Honor and Poetry in a Beduin Society*. Berkeley: University of California Press.

Adams, L. 2010. *The Spectacular Culture and National Identity in Uzbekistan*. Durham, N.C.: Duke University Press.

Akaev, A. 2003. *Kyrgyz Statehood and the Popular Epic 'Manas'*. Original in English.

Akiner, S. 1997. "Between Tradition and Modernity: The Dilemma Facing Contemporary Central Asian Women." In *Post-Soviet Women: From the Baltic to Central Asia*, edited by M. Buckley, 261–304. Cambridge: Cambridge University Press.

Appadurai, A. 1995. *The Social Life of Things: Commodities in Cultural Perspective*. Cambridge: Cambridge University Press.

Arendt, H. 1986. "Communicative Power." In *Power*, edited by S. Lukes, 59–74. New York: New York University Press.

Arendt, H. 1993 [1961]. *Between Past and Future: Eight Exercises in Political Thought*. London: Penguin Books.

Asad, T. 1983. *"The Idea of an Anthropology of Islam."* Occasional Papers. Washington DC: Center for Contemporary Arab Studies, Georgetown University.

Bailey, F. G. 1969. *Sratagems and Spoils: A Social Anthropology of Politics*. New York: Schocken.

Benda-Beckmann, F. von. 1979. *Property in Social Continuity. Continuity and Change in the Maintenance of Property Relationships Through Time in Minangkabau, West Sumatra*. The Hague: Martinus Nijhoff.

Berdymukhammedov, G. 2013. *Adamnama*.

Bergne, P. 2006. *The Birth of Tajikistan: National Identity and the Origins of the Republic*. London: I. B. Tauris.

Beyer, J. 2006. "Revitalisation, Invention and Continued Existence of the Kyrgyz Aksakal Courts: Listening to Pluralistic Accounts of History." *Dynamics of Plural Legal Orders. Special Double Issue, Journal of Legal Pluralism and Unofficial Law* 53–54 (2006), edited by F. von Benda-Beckmann and K. von Benda-Beckmann. , 141–76 Berlin: Lit.

Beyer, J. 2015. "Constitutional Faith: Law and Hope in Revolutionary Kyrgyzstan." *Ethnos. Journal of Anthropology* 80 (3): 320–345.

Beyer, J. 2016. *The Force of Custom: Law and the Ordering of Everyday Life in Kyrgyzstan*. Pittsburgh: University of Pittsburgh Press.

Billaud, J. 2015. *Kabul Carnival: Gender Politics in Postwar Afghanistan*. Philadelphia: University of Pennsylvania Press.

Blumer, H. 1969. *Symbolic Interaction: Perspective and Method*. Berkeley, CA: University of California Press.

Briggs, C. 1996. "The Politics of Discursive Authority in Research on the 'Invention of Tradition'." *Cultural Anthropology* 11 (4): 435–469.

Brubaker, R., M. Loveman, and P. Stamatov. 2004. "Ethnicity as Cognition." *Theory and Society* 33/1: 31–64.

Cleuziou, J., and L. Direnberger. (eds) 2016. "Gender and Nation in Post-Soviet Central Asia. From National Narratives to Women's Practices." *Nationalities Papers* 44 (2): 195–206.

Cocq, C. 2014. "Traditionalisation for Revitalisation: Tradition as a Concept and Practice in Contemporary Sámi Contexts." *Folklore* 57: 79–100.

Collins, K. 2007. "Ideas, Networks, and Islamist Movements. Evidence From Central Asia and the Caucasus." *World Politics* 60 (1): 64–96.

Comaroff, J., and J. Comaroff. 2009. *Ethnicity, Inc*. Chicaco: University of Chicago Press.

Commercio, M. 2015. "The Politics and Economics of 'Retraditionalization' in Kyrgyzstan and Tajikistan." *Post-Soviet Affairs* 31 (6): 529–556.

Dragadze, T. 1994. *'Islam in Azerbaijan and the Position of Women.' In Muslim Women's Choices. Religious Belief and Social Reality, Edited by C. Fawzi El-Solh and J. Mabro, 152–163*. Oxford: Berg.

Dubuisson, E. M. 2011. "Dialogic Authority: Kazakh Aitys Poets and Their Patrons." *Ethnographies of the State in Central Asia: Performing Politics*, edited by Madeleine Reeves, M. J. Rasanayagam and J. Beyer, 55—77. Bloomington: Indiana University Press.

Dubuisson, E.M. 2017. *Living Language. The Dialogic Emergence of an Ancestral Worldview*. Pittsburgh: University of Pittsburgh Press.

Dudoignon, S., and C. Noack, eds. 2014. *Allah's Kolkhozes: Migration, De-Stalinisation, Privatisation and the New Muslim Congregations in the Soviet Realm (1950s-2000s)*. Berlin: Klaus Schwarz.

Eisenstadt, S. N. 1973. "Post-Traditional Societies and the Continuity and Reconstruction of Tradition." *Daedalus* 102 (1): 1–28.

Eisenstadt, S.N. 2000. *Multiple Modernities. Daedalus* 129 (1): 1–29.

Ensminger, J. 1992. *Making a Market: The Institutional Transformation of an African Society. The Political Economy of Institutions and Decisions*. Cambridge, NY: Cambridge University Press.

Eriksen, T. 2007. *Globalization: The Key Concepts*. Berg: Oxford and New York.

Finke, P. 2004. *Nomaden im Transformationsprozess: Kasachen in der Post-Sozialistischen Mongolei.* Münster: Lit-Verlag.
Finke, P. 2014. *Variations on Uzbek Identity: Strategic Choices, Cognitive Schemas and Political Constraints in Identification Processes*. Oxford, NY: Berghahn Books.
Foucault, M. 1979. *Discipline and Punish: The Birth of the Prison*. New York: Vintage Books.
Garfinkel, H. 1967. *Studies in Ethnomethodology*. Englewood Cliffs, NJ: Prentice-Hall.
Geertz, C. 2000 [1983]. "Local Knowledge: Fact and Law in Comparative Perspective." In *Local Knowledge: Further Essays in Interpretive Anthropology*, edited by C. Geertz, 167–234. New York: Basic Books.
Girke, F. 2015. "The Uncertainty of Power and the Certainty of Irony: Encountering the State in Kara, Southern Ethiopia." In *Culture, Catastrophe, and Rhetoric: the Texture of Political Action*, edited by R. Hariman, and R. Cintron, 168–193. New York: Berghahn.
Glassie, H. 1995. "Tradition." *The Journal of American Folklore* 108 (430): 395–412.
Harris, C. 2004. *Control and Subversion: Gender Relations in Tajikistan*. London: Pluto.
Heathershaw, J. 2009. *Post-Conflict Tajikistan: The Politics of Peacebuilding and the Emergence of Legitimate Order*. London: Routledge.
Herzfeld, M. 2014 [2005]. *Cultural Intimacy: Social Poetics in the Nation-State*. London: Routledge.
Hirsch, F. 2005. *Empire of Nations: Ethnographic Knowledge and the Making of the Soviet Union*. Ithaca & London: Cornell University Press.
Hobsbawm, E., and T. Ranger. 1983. *The Invention of Tradition. Morgan Lectures Series*. Chicago: Aldine.
Hunn, E. 1993. "What is Traditional Ecological Knowledge?" In *Traditional Ecological Knowledge. Wisdom for Sustainable Development*, edited by N. Williams and G. Baines, 13-15. Canberra: Center for Resource and Environmental Studies, Australian National University.
Hutchinson, J. 1987. *The Dynamics of Cultural Nationalism: The Gaelic Revival and the Creation of the Irish Nation State*. Boston: Allen & Unwin.
Hutchinson, J. 1999. "Re-Interpreting Cultural Nationalism." *Australian Journal of Politics and History* 45 (3): 392–407.
Ismailbekova, A. 2016. "Constructing the Authority of Women Through Custom: Bulak Village, Kyrgyzstan." *Nationalities Papers* 44 (2): 266–280.
Ismailbekova, A. 2017. *Blood Ties and the Native Son Poetics of Patronage in Kyrgyzstan*. Bloomington: Indiana University Press.
Johnson, J., and J. Robinson, eds. 2006. *Living Gender After Communism*. Bloomington: Indiana University Press.
Jolly, M. 1992. "Specters of Inauthenticity." *The Contemporary Pacific* 4 (1): 49–72.
Jones Luong, P. 2002. *Institutional Change and Political Continuity in Post-Soviet Central Asia: Power, Perceptions, and Pacts*. Cambridge: Cambridge University Press.
Jones, P., ed. 2017. *Islam, Society and Politics in Central Asia*. Pittsburgh: Pittsburgh University Press.
Kamp, M. 2009. "Women's Studies and Gender Studies in Central Asia. Are We Talking to Each Other?" *Central Eurasian Studies Review* 8 (1): 2–12.
Kandiyoti, D. 1988. "Bargaining with Patriarchy." *Gender and Society* 2 (3): 274–290.
Kandiyoti, D. 2007. "Old Dilemmas, New Challenges: The Politics of Gender and Reconstruction in Afghanistan." *Development and Change* 28 (2): 169–199.
Karataev, O and S. Eraliev. 2005. *Kyrgyz Ethnografiiasy Boiuncha Sözdük*. Bishkek: Biiktik.
Karimov, I. 2008. *High Morality. An Invincible Force. [i.O. Yuksak Ma'naviyat - Yengilmas Kuch]*. Tashkent: Ma'naviyat.
Kassymbekova, B. 2017. "Understanding Stalinism in, from and of Central Asia." *Central Asian Survey* 36, 1: 1–18.
Kendzior, S. 2014. "Reclaiming Ma'naviyat. Morality, Criminalityand Dissident Politics in Uzbekistan." In *Ethnographies of the State in Central Asia. Performing Politics*, edited by M. Reeves, J. Rasanayagam and J. Beyer, 223-242. Bloomington: Indiana University Press.
Knight, J. 1992. *Institutions and Social Conflict. The Political Economy of Institutions and Decisions*. Cambridge, New York: Cambridge University Press.

Kocaoglu, T. 2009. "The Past as Prologue? Challenging the Myth of the Subordinate, Docile Woman in Muslim Central Eurasia." In *Gender Politics in Post-Communist Eurasia*, edited by L. Racioppi, and K. O'Sullivan, 169–208. East Lansing: Michigan State University Press.

Kroeber, A. 1948. *Anthropology: Race, Language, Culture*. New York: Hartcourt Brace.

Lukes, S. 2005 [1974]. *Power: A Radical View*. 2nd edition. Palgrave: Macmillan.

Lukes, S., ed. 1986. *Power*. New York: New York University Press.

Martin, V. 2001. *Law and Custom in the Steppe. The Kazakhs of the Middle Horde and Russian Colonialism in the Nineteenth Century*. Surrey, England: Curzon Press.

Massell, G. 1975. "Family Law and Social Mobilization in Soviet Central Asia. Some Comparisons with Socialist China." *Canadian Slavonic Papers* 17: 374–403.

McGlinchey, E. 2009. *Chaos, Violence, Dynasty: Politics and Islam in Central Asia*. Pittsburgh: University of Pittsburgh Press.

McGuire, G. 2017. "Cultural Histories of Kumiss: Tuberculosis, Heritage and National Health in Post-Soviet Kazakhstan." *Central Asian Survey* 36/4: 493–510.

Megoran, N. 1999. "Theorizing Gender, Ethnicity and the Nation-State in Central Asia." *Central Asian Survey* 18 (1): 99–110.

Morozova, I. 2005. "Nation-Building in Central Asia: Creating New State Mythologies." In *Towards Social Stability and Democratic Governance in Central Eurasia*, edited by I. Morozova. *NATO Science Series, V: Science and Technology Policy* 49: 67–81. Oxford: IOS Press.

Mould, T. 2005. "The Paradox of Traditionalization: Negotiating the Past in Choctaw Prophetic Discourse." *Journal of Folklore Research* 42 (3): 255–294.

Munkh-Erdene, E. 2008. "Selling of Good Father's Name: Legitimacy, Pride and Commodity. Commemoration of Chinggis Khan in Modern Mongolia." *Bulletin* 24: 35–36.

Nazarbaev, N. 2001. *Epicenter of Peace*. Hollis, NH: Puritan Press.

Nazarbaev, N. 2008. *The Kazakhstan Way*. London: Stacey International.

North, D. 1990. *Institutions, Institutional Change, and Economic Performance: The Political Economy of Institutions and Decisions*. Cambridge, New York: Cambridge University Press.

Northrop, D. 2004. *Veiled Empire. Gender and Power in Stalinist Central Asia*. Ithaca, NY: Cornell University Press.

Noyes, D. 2009. "Tradition: Three Traditions." *Journal of Folklore Research* 46 (3): 233–268.

Nyazov, S. 2005 [2001]. *Rukhnama: Reflections on the Spiritual Values of the Turkmen*. Ashgabat: State Publishing Service Turkmenistan.

Paskaleva, E. 2016. *Memory and Commemoration in Central Asia*. IIAS Newsletter 74. Online: http://www.iias.asia/sites/default/files/IIAS_NL74_FULL.pdf (accessed 20 August 2017).

Peabody, R. L. 1968. "Authority." In *International Encyclopedia of the Social Sciences 1*, edited by D. L. Sills, and R. K. Merton, 473–474. New York: Macmillan/Free Press.

Pelkmans, M. 2017. *Fragile Conviction: Changing Ideological Landscapes in Urban Kyrgyzstan*. Ithaca and London: Cornell University Press.

Penkala-Gawecka, D. 2013. "Mentally Ill Or Chosen By Spirits? 'Shamanic Illness' and the Revival Of Kazakh Traditional Medicine in Post-Soviet Kazakhstan." *Central Asian Survey* 32 (1): 37–51.

Rahmon, E. 2009 [2001]. *Tochikon dar Oinai Tar'ikh. Kitobi Iakum, Az Orien to Somonien*. Dushanbe: Irfon.

Ranger, T. 1993. 'The Invention of Tradition Revisited: The Case of Colonial Africa' Legitimacy and the State in the Twentieth-Century Africa, edited by Terence Ranger and Olufemi Vaughan, 62–111: Springer.

Rasanayagam, J. 2011. *Islam in Post-Soviet Uzbekistan: The Morality of Experience*. Cambridge: Cambridge University Press.

Rasanayagam, J. 2014. "The Politics of Culture and the Space for Islam: Soviet and Post-Soviet Imaginaries in Uzbekistan." *Central Asian Survey* 33 (1): 1–14.

Reeves, M. 2010. "Migrations, Masculinité et Transformations de L'espace Social Dans la Vallée de Sokh." In *Dynamiques Migratoires et Changements Sociétaux en Asie Centrale*, edited by M. Laruelle, 131–147. Paris: Editions Petra.

Roche, S. 2014. *Domesticating Youth: Youth Bulges and Their Socio-Political Implications in Tajikistan*. New York and Oxford: Berghahn.

Roy, O. 2000. *The New Central Asia: The Creation of Nations*. London: I. B. Tauris.
Sahlins, M. 1999. "'Two or Three Things That I Know About Culture.' Huxley Lecture 1998." *Journal of the Royal Anthropological Institute* 5: 399–421.
Schröder, P. 2017. *Bishkek Boys: Neighbourhood Youth and Urban Change in Kyrgyzstan's Capital*. New York and Oxford: Berghahn.
Scott, J. 1987. *Weapons of the Weak. Everyday Forms of Peasant Resistance*. New Haven: Yale University Press.
Strauss, C., and N. Quinn. 1997. *A Cognitive Theory of Cultural Meaning*. Cambridge, New York: Cambridge University Press.
Tabyshalieva, A. 2000. "Revival of Traditions in Post-Soviet Central Asia." *Making the transition work for women in Europe and Central* Asia, edited by Marina Lazreg, 51–57. World Bank Discussion Paper No 411. Washington, DC.
Tett, G. 1994. "Guardians of the Faith? Gender and Religion in an (ex) Soviet Tajik Village." In *Muslim Women's Choices. Religious Belief and Social Reality*, edited by C. Fawzi El-Solh, and J. Mabro, 128–151. Oxford: Berg.
Thibault, H. 2017. "Labour Migration, Sex, And Polygyny: Negotiating Patriarchy in Tajikistan." *Ethnic and Racial Studies*. Published online first: https://doi.org/10.1080/01419870.2017.1400086.
Vuillemenot, A.-M. 2009. *La Yourte et la Mesure du Monde: Avec les Nomades au Kazakhstan*. Louvain-la-Neuve: Academia.
Wagner, R. 1975. *The Invention of Culture*. Englewoods Cliffs, NJ: Prentice-Hall.
Weber, M. 1922. "Die Drei Reinen Typen der Legitimen Herrschaft." *Preussische Jahrbücher* 187 (1): 1–12.
Werner, C. 2009. "Bride Abduction in Post-Soviet Central Asia: Marking a Shift Towards Patriarchy Through Local Discourses of Shame and Tradition." *Journal of the Royal Anthropological Institute* 15 (2): 314–331.
Wolf, E. 1999. *Envisioning Power: Ideologies of Dominance and Crisis*. Berkeley, CA et al.: University of California Press.
Yuval-Davis, N. 1997. *Gender and Nation*. London: Sage.
Zanca, R. 2003. "Take! Take! Take! Host-Guest Relations and All That Food: Uzbek Hospitality Past and Present." *Anthropology of East Europe Review* 21 (1): 8–16.

Women of protest, men of applause: political activism, gender and tradition in Kyrgyzstan

Judith Beyer and Aijarkyn Kojobekova

ABSTRACT

Tradition has come to play an important role throughout Central Asia in a number of new ways since independence, but has been predominantly investigated regarding nation building. In this article, we show how tradition is being used operationally in the context of activism and political conflict. We expose the various motivations and tactics pursued by aksakals (lit., whitebeards) and by a movement of mature women called OBON (lit., Women Units for Special Purposes) as they participate in politics, and the role tradition plays in these activities. We argue that aksakals actively draw on tradition even in the political realm to avoid being derogatorily labelled 'elders on duty', whereas OBON women position themselves as economic and political actors but are subjected to discourses and practices of tradition by others. While both aksakals and OBON women have been central to political action in Kyrgyzstan in the last two decades, this article is the first to compare and contrast these two categories of unusual activists. The comparison reveals a perpetuation of culturally recognized gender roles even when these actors go beyond their 'traditional' realms of competence.

Introduction

Often considered the most democratic of Central Asian countries, Kyrgyzstan has a highly volatile political landscape. Since its independence in 1991, its citizens have witnessed, taken part in or protested against changes in government, regular parliamentary and presidential elections, and several constitutional referenda. These political developments have been widely analysed with emphases on institution building, party politics, corruption, local manifestations of the state, 'tribalism' and democracy.[1] Although in Kyrgyzstan 'the level of political activism is high, and opposition groups and citizens have been quick to protest government policies related to corruption, human rights abuses, and the environment' (Engvall 2015, 1), we are still lacking in-depth investigations of political activism, its emergence, its different formats and its (inner) workings.

While political activism is usually studied from the perspective of social movements (e.g., Hardtmann 2017) with a focus on goal realization, agenda-setting, or the management of resources (Acosta 2018), participation in the type of political activism we are concerned with in this article is motivated by individual interests but realized and recognized through the embodiment and enactment of public collective personae. Thus, we investigate and compare the roles of male elders (*aksakals*, lit. whitebeards) as well as mature women, the latter often derogatorily referred to as OBON (Women's Units for Special Purposes[2]), in the context of political activism and political conflict. Both types of activists have moved beyond what are generally considered their 'traditional' realms of competence: the village and the lineage, and the household and family, respectively. We also demonstrate that their performances are in different ways enabled and constrained by practices and discourses of tradition that play a central role in the political arena in Kyrgyzstan. Their activities complement (rather than oppose) conventional party politics: they can in one context be seen as supporting 'the state' while in another they may challenge state officials. In any case, the performances of these actors speak of an emerging awareness of what agentic engagement by citizens can achieve (Meyer and Jepperson 2000).

In this article, we approach the concept of tradition from a praxeological perspective, asking how tradition is demonstrated, claimed, negotiated and put to use by local actors themselves. Methodologically, we consider tradition an interpretative concept that always needs to be analysed from a concrete empirical situation. When actors invoke something as traditional, they engage in an act of sense-making in which they align their own actions with the expectations of others. If successful, the invocation of tradition might lend authority or at least legitimacy to an individual's behaviour (or the behaviour of people aggregated into a group persona), which then becomes recognized and categorized by others as appropriate, as in the case of the aksakals. However, this does not mean that tradition necessarily harmonizes social relationships; it can also affirm power asymmetries, as inequality can be legitimized through the successful invocation of tradition. This is the case for OBON women, who want to be recognized as economic and political actors, but are generally characterized and subsequently dismissed for 'acting like women' in the first place. We will argue, however, that this portrayal also allows for their very political participation in protest movements because it complements the aksakals: these mature women can behave in ways male elders cannot, and they have come to use their 'traditional' gendered roles in new and innovative ways. It is therefore of interest to politicians to engage both types of actors for their political gains.

Elders and women in politics

In 2005, Kyrgyzstan went through its Tulip Revolution, which began in the southern part of the country and led to an overthrow of the government (Pelkmans 2005; Cummings and Ryabkov 2008; Cummings 2010). In reflecting on this event, Knyazev positions two unusual types of political activists alongside each other without, however, elaborating on what brings them together in political action. He writes, 'On 18 March, the building of the oblast administration in Osh was seized. First horsemen broke through the police cordon, and then, *elders and women* went into the gangway' (Knyazev 2005, 95, cited in Temirkulov 2010, 99; emphasis added). The fact that (male) 'elders' and 'women' (who are denied a specific respectful label in the report) were at the forefront of political action reflects a recent trend whereby the two types of actors have become crucial to Kyrgyzstan's activist landscape. This juxtaposition of *elders and women* brings the role of age and gender in political activism to our attention: What do these categories afford, and how do they constrain? In the following, we pursue a comparative investigation of gendered and age-based activism in the light of traditional expectations.

The first group of activists we investigate are the elderly men known as aksakals. The stereotypical depiction of an aksakal is of a long-bearded man, wearing a gold-embroidered *chapan* (coat or robe) and a *kalpak* (a white felt hat). Before the Russian conquest of Central Asia, aksakals served as mediators in cases of conflict and presided over their lineages. Aksakals from different lineages would gather in councils (*kurultais*) to discuss problems and conflicts. When the Russian government began its administrative and territorial reorganization of Central Asia in the nineteenth century, aksakal became an elected position in the villages or encampments, with the elected elders being put in charge of collecting taxes. The earlier ad hoc character of the council was turned into a 'people's court' (Russ.: *narodnyi sud*) during Soviet times and, as such, lost its informality and flexibility (Edgar 2004; Brusina 2005). After independence, most Central Asian nations employed aksakals in their nation-building efforts in the form of consultative, administrative or even judicial institutions. Beyer (2005, 2006, 2014a) in particular has researched their roles in various social, political and legal arenas, such as in the aksakal courts in the countryside and the capital Bishkek (Beyer 2015), in their position as *bash* (lit., head) representing their households or heading their lineages (*eng uluu aksakal*; Beyer 2010, 2016), and in their efforts to form new local institutions (Beyer 2014b). There are fleeting references to the political activism of aksakals, for example when (Reeves 2014, 209) writes that in her field site in southern Batken Province 'elders petitioned the regional governor to remove the Kyrgyz border post altogether, and asked that the water allocation schedule which had existed prior to 2002 be reinstated', or when Bichsel (2009) describes the manifold roles elders have when it comes to local dispute resolution in the Fergana Valley.[3] However, despite their public visibility, aksakals' active interventions in public and political life have thus far received little attention. It has also not been sufficiently analysed how their stereotypical depiction as 'traditional authorities' who are wise and worthy of respect translates into social practice that enables them to legitimately act in the public arena.

The second group of activists we are concerned with are collectively referred to as OBON, which, as noted above, is an acronym for a Russian phrase that can be translated as Women's Units for Special Purposes. This label was introduced in reference to mature women, usually in their forties and fifties, who organized and participated in demonstrations and protests during the 2005 Tulip Revolution and the 2010 *coup d'état* that led to another overthrow of the government. Their motivations can be related to wider social problems in Kyrgyzstan, such as unemployment and poverty, but they have also issued demands that concern the just distribution of land, material security, and recognition in the political arena, as we elaborate in this article.

Satybaldieva (2018) has noted that post-Soviet gender discourses have generally tended to view women as politically inactive (see also Kocaoglu 2009), but it is possible that this characterization is due to a lack of studies of their grass-roots activism. While there is a wide range of reports and initiatives from international non-governmental organizations, sometimes in tandem with state institutions, to investigate, strengthen and protect women's rights, those rights have often been seen merely as means to advance other goals, such as democratization, the establishment of human rights measures more generally, or 'to prevent potential ethnic and sub-ethnic conflicts in local communities' (Hasanov, Biybosunova, and Hasanova 2009, 33). In response to such campaigns, which are often foreign-funded and top-down in their approach, scholars have more recently started to investigate women's struggles for acknowledgement of their agency in public arenas on their own terms. Drawing on Kandiyoti's (1988, 279) argument of the 'patriarchal bargain', according to which Central Asian women have internalized a form of patriarchy by accepting that their power lies within the sphere of their households, Ismailbekova (2016, 278) has shown that in contemporary Kyrgyzstan, the ideology of women as 'privileged custodians of national values' (note the strong conflation of the trope of woman-as-nurturer and tradition) helps hide the fact that 'the state cannot successfully manage its paternalistic tasks'. In this manner, women's authority has been shown to extend beyond the private and into the public realm. Spector (2017, 147) has shown how *baibiche* – a term she translates as 'respected older women' and which refers to female traders in Bishkek's Osh bazaar – mediate 'disputes between traders and clients, or between traders and the bazaar administration'. Spector positions the baibiche alongside the aksakals, who also serve in a similar role at the bazaar. Beyond reports of individual women assuming positions of political authority,[4] accounts such as Spector's, which indicate where women can – *qua* women – collectively or categorically exert agency outside the domestic sphere, suggest that a social innovation is afoot. Satybaldieva (2018, 261) has investigated OBON activities in Kyrgyzstan more concretely, portraying OBON women as strategic actors who not only manage to achieve their economic goals, but who also critique gender norms in the process, thereby transforming 'feelings of shame and humiliation about debt and homelessness into ideas of entitlements and rights'.

We intend to contribute to and expand this emerging literature by arguing that *both* elderly men and women who participate in political activism in contemporary Kyrgyzstan are assigned to culturally accepted gender roles by third parties and engage elements of a cultural model of tradition. This shows that such actors are not necessarily the unwitting subjects of traditionalization. To the contrary, our empirical material reveals strategic, creative and often contradictory ways in which tradition is brought into play by the actors themselves.

Of whitebeards and warriors

In everyday Kyrgyz life, the duty of aksakals is often 'to sit' at festive occasions, marking these as socially proper and in line with tradition. During such events, aksakals are asked to give blessings (*bata*), and it is through their well-wishing that events are rendered legitimate and 'orderly'. These practices occur during life-cycle celebrations such as births, weddings and anniversaries, as well as at funerals and mourning rituals. The 'sitting' of aksakals can also be encountered during annual rituals such as spring festivals, and particularly on Veterans' Day, commemorated throughout the country on 9 May. The elders' accepted and expected role is to publicly display the wisdom they are perceived as embodying. The proverb 'a beard is needed at a feast' (Kyrg.: *sakal toido kerek*) conveys the respect that people accord aksakals and the expectations people have of them.

Ambitious young men tap into such traditional imagery to lend credibility to their efforts to rise to positions of authority. In the last decade in particular, we have witnessed an increase in symbols in the public arena that are commonly understood as 'traditionally Kyrgyz'. The nationalist movement Kyrk Choro (40 Warriors), for example, named itself in reference to the 40 warriors who – according to myth – formed the backbone of the Kyrgyz when they arrived in what is present-day Kyrgyzstan.[5] According to Niiazova (2015), the movement counts some 5000 members. It has eight regional representatives in each province, as well as in Bishkek, its own charter, a seal, and is registered with the Ministry of Justice, which demonstrates its interlinkage with the state apparatus. It is also said to have significant overlaps with organized crime. Since 2010 Kyrk Choro members have become notorious throughout the country for their objections to women's 'untraditional' behaviour and for beating up prostitutes and women who are in relationships with foreigners. They have also inspected village shops and market stalls to find out if alcohol was being sold there.

Within such movements, but also among young, ambitious political candidates across the political spectrum, it is common nowadays to sport kalpaks, the Kyrgyz felt hats, which only a few years ago were worn almost exclusively by aksakals, as many of Beyer's aksakal interlocutors emphasized. The kalpak has, in their perception at least, shifted from a visible sign of authority to an ostentatious symbol of nationalism and male pride (see also Suyarkulova 2016). During the presidential elections in 2017, for example, all the candidates wore *kalpaks* on the campaign trail, when speaking in public, and in the photographs that graced the banners and posters advertising their candidacy throughout the country.[6] The degree to which the kalpak has become a *pars pro toto* for Kyrgyz national identity was revealed in December 2017, when a dog in a dog show in Bishkek was paraded around wearing a kalpak. One parliamentarian scoffed, 'We put our national symbol on a dog. They turned a dog into a Kyrgyz, and a Kyrgyz into a dog.' Another was quoted saying that the state prosecuting attorney should look into the issue, as 'the pride of the country' was at stake.[7]

While nationalists and politicians have thus appropriated the kalpak, which is no longer understood primarily as an accessory of elders but more as an expression of commitment to tradition, whose misuse can trigger accusations, politicians are still in need of the elders' presence at political rallies. There, aksakals are offered food and often receive presents, cash and applause as markers of the 'respect' they command. The elders' presence lends legitimacy to the politicians' causes, as they become aligned with figures associated with upholding and embodying tradition. The politicians thus mimic expected behaviour towards elders in the realm of the family, household or lineage.

But the relationship is more mutual still: politicians are generally referred to as heads (*bash*) in Kyrgyz society, and aksakals accordingly demonstrate that they, too, respect these political leaders, even if they are much younger and – in a traditional view – not the equals of a proper elder. The events in which such mutual acknowledgment takes place are mediatized, with TV stations broadcasting these acts of recognition widely. Usually it is the elders' mere presence that is demanded, and they are not even asked to publicly voice an opinion, but at times they are also asked to give speeches in support of a political candidate or – more frequently – of those already in power. It is on such occasions that they invoke notions such as harmony (*yntymak*) and calm or peacefulness (*tynchtyk*) as prerequisites for enabling the incumbent politicians to carry out their work for the people. Elders will recite proverbs and draw on shared narratives to speak in parables, and in general offer formalized speech acts with an emphasis on tradition. These aspects were also characteristic of talks given by rural elders that Beyer recorded during her research in the Talas region.

In April 2006, for example, an aksakal war veteran gave the following speech in support of the sitting governor of Talas Province, who had invited around 15 elders from different parts of the province to the main square in front of the White House (the seat of the local government) to discuss how to prevent turmoil during the upcoming parliamentary elections:

> Let's be peaceful and help each other. Let's be united. If parents have good behaviour, children will also behave properly.... If people scream at each other, a conflict will start. Nowadays young people don't listen to old people. Long ago if there was a boy doing something bad, people would invite an aksakal like me and ask him to talk to him. The aksakal would say: 'Come here, who is your father?' 'I am the son of this person.' 'You did this bad thing. Stop it!' And the boy would stop. Are you [addressing absent politicians of the opposition, accused of sowing discord] behaving like this now? If your sons are outside all day, how can you tell? You don't know, right? Even if they are smoking, you don't tell us [aksakals]. But can you tell? Of course, you can. Why wouldn't they stop? They will stop! ... Let Kyrgyzstan be peaceful. Let's be united and be far away from bad things. Let's not disturb [former president] Bakiev in his work and give him a chance to work. Let's be united. This is what I wanted to say.

Invoking a distant past in which the young listened to the old, the aksakal first appealed to the audience's consciousness of having to cherish one's ancestors and the traditional way of Kyrgyz life. While admitting that respect towards elders was waning, the aksakal also showcased his authority by declaring that young people would of course 'stop' if only they were told to. He then aligned the respect that should be accorded elders with a situation of overall peace in the country, which in turn he suggested the president needed in order to 'work' properly.

While the default stance of aksakals is that of supporting incumbent state officials, some have also supported opposition candidates by emphasizing their personal relationships, referring to them as 'my good child' who knows how to respect his parents and who is doing good things for 'his people' (see also Ismailbekova 2017). Such staged political rallies that invoke tradition can of course be contrasted with the common complaint of ordinary citizens that it is precisely those politicians who engage in such activities who are not acting in accordance with tradition.

In any case, the contribution of aksakals thus appears to be fundamental to political rallies, as it difficult to demand allegiance, display patriotism and claim a leadership role without invoking tradition. Hence, government officials continue to clothe their policies and personae in legitimacy and an ideology of harmony (Beyer and Girke 2015) by surrounding themselves with elders while denying their opponents' claims to that selfsame legitimacy and reassuring connection with tradition. During these events, state officials and elders collude in the spectacle of speaking in the name of tradition. While there is sometimes unwanted pressure on the elders to comply with the summons of officials and adhere to the procedure of 'being invited', the actual form of the meetings has also become a welcome occasion to display their aksakal-ness to others. Respect and authority do not come automatically with a certain age, but must be earned through interaction with others who recognize one's performance as adequate and worthy of an aksakal. In a larger setting, this might not require much effort for an individual aksakal; the embodiment of a certain dignified manner is generally enough to pass muster. Elders thus seek moments in which they can publicly display those qualities that are generally attributed to 'whitebeards'. These practices can best be understood as co-emergent products of joint performances, and they extend established tropes and imagery to a relatively innovative setting and social arrangement.

Troubled women causing trouble?

In Kyrgyzstan, there is no female equivalent to the aksakals when it comes to public visibility and the wide range of private and public performative tasks in everyday life. There is the figure of Umai Ene, the spiritual mother of birth, who is represented during public celebrations such as Nowruz (spring festival) and who might be co-opted for political purposes, as, for example, when she helped symbolically 'free' the Kyrgyz constitution from 'evil forces' in the aftermath of the March revolution of 2005 (Beyer 2015). But she provides no everyday counterpart to the manifold roles of the aksakals. In contrast to Soviet times (Bridger 1987; Attwood 1999; Kandiyoti 2007), in the last decade women in Kyrgyzstan have been increasingly erased from public representation. They are rarely given visible space or tasks in public life: politics has become an almost entirely male endeavour.[8] In 2011, the prominent winged female statue of Liberty (Erkindik) on one of Bishkek's central squares was replaced by the warrior figure of the national hero, Manas.[9] The female statue had held the centrepiece of a yurt (a *tündük*) up to the sky – a combination that was denounced as untraditional and even dangerous.[10] At the same time, one of the most watched and debated reality shows in contemporary Kyrgyzstan is *Kelin* (lit.: daughter-in-law), in which a number of young women have to prove themselves worthy before a potential mother-in-law (*kain-ene*) who judges their skills in serving tea, handicrafts and the like. The prize is advertised as 'dowry' and includes furniture and a trip to Turkey. The show has been criticized for its sexism and clichéd portrayal of women in Kyrgyz society (Iskender 2017), but it is indicative of an intensification of traditionalization that assigns a stereotypically gendered role to women. This sort of representation also excludes the very idea of women's collective action – women's relations are either limited to their respective domestic domain or greatly abstracted as motherhood or daughter-in-law status, subordinated to other roles in the family, or at least defined by others. There is no traditional way in which women can form corporate bodies that might act in public.[11]

Given this context, the emergence of a public movement of women (which came to be called OBON) in Kyrgyzstan from 2005 onwards is striking; at a time when there were no women in parliament, there were many in the streets. Was it this public representational gap that stimulated the emergence of OBON as an alternative space in which women could engage and be heard? Most people in Kyrgyzstan associate OBON with women who engage in political protest: they participate in demonstrations, march along with the crowd, speak into microphones, and even shout out slogans. This behaviour would be considered fully in line with encouraged civil activity in a democracy, yet its portrayal in both local and international media is mostly negative, and the public image of these women is likewise less than respectable.[12] Depictions focus on displays of aggressive behaviour against opponents, screaming, cursing and even physical attacks. While one may argue that their activities as organized protestors clearly go against what would be considered traditional female behaviour, their transgressions of traditional values still rely on other aspects commonly associated with the stereotypical female: being loud and gossipy in general, and 'causing trouble' to get their message across and to achieve their personal goals.

These tactics were successfully used in the streets during the 2005 Tulip Revolution, when they were first labelled OBON. After 2005, more protesting women made visible appearances during the 2007 parliamentary election campaign and the 2010 *coup d'état*, and were labelled OBON as well. Most of the women who were seen participating were in their forties or fifties; observers would accordingly assume that the OBON women had children, and that many might be single mothers or widows, who often carry an economic burden and face social stigmatization.[13] In our research we found that state officials and NGO workers as a rule considered most of the women who participated in 'OBON activities' socially and financially vulnerable; their participation, therefore, was assumed to have been bought cheaply by patrons who stayed in the background. This rendering of the women's motivation already de-emphasizes their agency and genuine political aspirations, which, we argue, often grew out of their vulnerable situation. And the very act of calling these women OBON attributes a corporate identity to a diffuse social form that cannot *a priori* be assumed to be an organized group with card-carrying 'members' or an official 'agenda'. In their 'Alternative Report to the Fourth Periodic Report of the Kyrgyz Republic to the CEDAW Committee', the Council of NGOs in Kyrgyzstan (2014) described OBON as follows:

> OBON is an established informal group, consisting mainly [of] women, purposefully formed and valid for the purposes of specific customers (government and other political structures, business, semi-criminal elements), regularly applying aggressive, violent, and illegal methods of work. OBON does not belong to true civil society groups, as it neither represents [its] own interests or the interests of vulnerable groups.

Beyond the obvious uncertainty about the status of the women, as evidenced by the awkward juxtaposition of 'established' and 'informal', the report further states that any OBON-related activity would hamper women's 'real' political participation. It was true that OBON supported other people's agendas: our research indicates that businessmen and political candidates bent on hiring OBON women after 2005 apparently had access to lists of people who had already participated in a previous protest. Such lists were even stored at some party offices. Alternatively, campaigners needing to recruit marchers could try to gain access to official data on socially vulnerable women from village administrations or city townships. Patrons without direct access to this type of data could thus buy it from department heads or local administrative staff. At the same time, interviews with state personnel and NGO workers revealed a deep mistrust of women's motives for joining such activities. But though they were accused of being 'in it for the money', the perspective of the women themselves was different. Medina, for example, emphasized her difficult economic situation as a motivating factor:

> I used to work in many different places, as a dishwasher or a cleaner. I only have secondary education. I got married very early and never continued my education. I could hardly manage to earn enough money to buy something good for my kids. Cleaners are not paid well despite the hard work, and people usually despise us. They treat us awfully, as if we were not human beings. I had been struggling to survive for several years since my husband left me. He does not help us at all. (Medina, 42 years old in 2015)[14]

Another woman in her early forties, who now works in the mayor's office as head of the department for social work, argued as follows:

> Our women live a very hard life. They do not have a lot of opportunities like men do. Some of them do not know where to direct their leadership skills. Local authorities should try to understand them, teach them, help them. But instead of that they call them OBON. ... I saw that there were a lot of very smart and active women, but they have no opportunities to participate in public life. Some of them asked me to help them somehow. They knew that I had always been very active. I know that some colleagues of mine think that I am *obonovka* [a member of OBON], but I just let active women express their opinions, demand from the authorities what they need. (Aitolkun, 42 years old in 2015)

The way Aitolkun put it reveals that women's political activism is often motivated by a lack of economic security and by the difficult situation mothers (particularly single mothers) find themselves in. While some women with whom Kojobekova spoke admitted to needing the money that was offered to them as a one-time payment, from 2008 onwards new incentives were available that went beyond the immediate payment for attending and performing at demonstrations. Patrons who had relied on women's performances in their political campaigns and had been successful were pressured by the women to give them administrative positions such as head of a local kindergarten, school or NGO, or positions in village administrations (*aiyl ökmötü*), or even regional state offices (*akimat*) and township councils (*mikroraion*, TOS). The women sometimes also insisted on the promotion of relatives to such positions. Some women who had participated in both the revolution of 2005 and the 2010 *coup d'état* even received land or apartments. As a consequence, others argued that they only started to copy the 'aggressive behaviour' they had witnessed in other women once it became clear that those women managed to have their demands met. A woman in her fifties who is now heading a local NGO said:

> I, along with other women from my village, demanded land for our families, too. We saw that some very aggressive, impudent women [Russ.: *aggressivnye naglye zhenshchiny*] had received land plots after they organized protests against the village administration. I also wanted to have land for my children. Who knows what will be? Land is always important. So, yes, we went to the mayor and we demanded land. Of course, they did not want to give us anything, but why should we pay when we were born here and have been working here all our lives? I think we had a right to get land. But I am not like these women who are participating in all possible protests just to be paid. I participated only in the meetings for land while other women wanted a change of powers. I believed that it [what I did] was right. (Aidai, 52 years old in 2015)

Here as well, the motivation to join protest actions was articulated by way of an analogy to a mother who has to take care of her children. Pure economic motivation was denied, and instead a discourse of rights was foregrounded that Aidai and others felt entitled to as citizens. It is important to note that the aggressive behaviour that has become so characteristic of OBON activities is here explicitly referenced as a performative strategy and linked to a higher probability of realizing economic gains and/or exercising one's political agency. A Russian woman in her forties who in 2015 was also a member of an NGO argued as follows:[15]

> I know that our administration calls me OBON because I am very active [Russ.: *aktivnaia*]. I want to influence situations – I cannot be indifferent [Russ.: *Ia ne mogu byt' ravnodushnoi*]. If we do

> not demand something, our authorities will do nothing. They want us to be stupid, passive and not to cause trouble for them. But we do not make trouble, we merely ask them to do their jobs. ... OBON in the eyes of the authorities are those who know their rights. ... One could say that all members of our local NGOs might be called OBON because we demand a lot from them [laughs].

The hurdles faced by women in Kyrgyzstan trying to collectively work towards better services and access are apparent: if they do not cause 'trouble', they will not be heard; if they do cause trouble, they might be heard, but will at the same time be delegitimized as political actors. While the stereotypical depiction of women had been to 'not cause trouble', and thus, one could argue, was very much in line with how the state tends to employ the presence and performances of aksakals in the political arena, we can see that women take the negative depiction of their activism and turn it into the positive characterization of an empowered female citizen, a view that they then cleverly attribute to state officials rather than to themselves.

Of elders on duty and shameless women

Explicit public endorsement of parties and policies ('talking or performing politics') is considered improper behaviour for aksakals and women, as both are traditionally understood to act in and for the lineage and/or the house. But members of both categories have nevertheless become a familiar type of collective actor in the recent political history of Kyrgyzstan. Although the elders' performances are officially apolitical, and they purportedly act only according to tradition, the instrumentality of their performances is rather apparent. They therefore need to carefully set off their behaviour from 'dirty politics' if they want to avoid being called an 'elder on duty' (*dezhurnyi chal*) – a derogatory term used for undeserving aksakals who seek profit and police others. The combination of the Russian adjective *dezhurnyi* (on duty) with the Kyrgyz word for old man (*chal*) hints at the origins of this concept in Soviet or even tsarist times, when elders were first approached in their roles as heads or mediators by Russian officials. The difference between an elder speaking about *yntymak* and an elder giving a speech in what informants termed the 'Soviet style' (Russ.: *po sovetski*[16]) became very clear to Beyer when she witnessed an aksakal standing bolt upright in front of the microphone, talking very loudly about the political chaos in the country, praising the president (or governor of the province), and ending the speech by shouting 'Hurrah!' Some elders in the audience laughingly responded with 'Hurrah!' and applauded his speech. Most others just laughed about the anachronistic performance, and it was not entirely clear whether those who had answered 'Hurrah!' were also making fun of the elder's misjudgement in terms of the time and the occasion, or whether they, being reminded of former times, genuinely approved of his performance.

To dissociate the aksakals' performances from the protests and demonstrations of opposition forces, often referred to by the English word 'meetings' (*miting*), events that endorse the status quo are referred to locally as 'anti-meetings' (Russ./Kyrg.: *antimiting*). When in April 2006 the incumbent governor of Talas Province invited aksakals to join him on stage, as described earlier in this article, members of the audience characterized the ongoing event to Beyer as such an *antimiting*. In his speech, while acknowledging that all 75 parliamentary seats would be taken by 'our brave men', the governor was nevertheless eager to warn of the seeds of discord that would be sown if the political opposition were to find their way into parliament:

> Because of one mandate, they are ready to destroy the Kyrgyz people by distributing vodka to every household – or is it a lie? They divided a father from a son. They divided a wife from a husband. They divided us into lineages, relatives and regions. Who are these people? Some deputies!

The aksakals nodded their heads and some of them applauded. The governor then began to address the elders specifically:

> Long ago in my village, I was small but I remember it, aksakals taught us not to spit into the flowing water. I think people of my age know about this. We listened and did not spit. We used to hide from aksakals when we smoked. And what is it like now? If an aksakal speaks, people call him an aksakal on duty [*dezhurnyi aksakal*]. We stopped respecting elders. This is a sign of faith [*yiman*] fading away. Dear young people, we cannot improve Kyrgyzstan unless we become patriots of our country. We will never ever be able to develop Kyrgyzstan if we run after one piece of meat, selling our Motherland for it, supporting an Englishman [foreigner], or picketing and blocking roads.

His example of how the youth used to respect aksakals and how they are no longer doing so was sandwiched between his complaints about politicians dividing society and citizens lacking patriotism, culminating in the accusation that those who protest betray their country.

While aksakals do not usually voice any unease when appearing at political events and none ever expressed worry about being labelled a *dezhurnyi chal* to either author, the authors found that their female informants frequently mentioned the danger of an accusation of shameful behaviour. Women who were recruited by male patrons or more senior women were aware that their involvement was ethically problematic, but pursued it nonetheless:

> I earned 500 *som* just for standing in the square with other women.[17] I was ashamed [Kyrg.: *Men zhaman uialyp turdum*] at the beginning and just tried to be as invisible as possible. Then I was told that if I am able to convince other women to protest, I will be paid for each of them separately. I have never earned so much money in such a short amount of time. (Jarmila, 42 years old in 2015)

Despite some initial misgivings, over the years Jarmila has come to terms with her activities:

> People think that in OBON only crazy women [Kyrg.: *esi zhok katyndar*, lit. hags with no brains] participate, but we are not crazy; we just want to feed our children. It is also work, but not like usual work. It is also hard. And we are paid for doing this. On the one hand, I cannot respect myself [Kyrg.: *cyimyktanbaim*] for doing this kind of work, but on the other hand, I do respect myself [Kyrg.: *cyimyktanganga*] because I am not stealing anything; I am not killing anybody – I earn bread for my children.

In admitting that she had been 'scared', Jarmila signalled that she understood from the beginning that her involvement in OBON would be frowned upon. But she rejected the public attribution of women acting 'crazy' by juxtaposing this portrayal with her duty as a mother feeding her children. This, she argued, was her final motivation for joining protest activities – something of which she was 'proud' now. She thus reinterpreted her behaviour to make it compatible with traditional expectations of women in Kyrgyz society, that is, being good mothers (compare Ismailbekova 2016). That she was 'ashamed' and rejected the attribute 'crazy' points to a connected emotional discourse that centres on women's modesty and moral conscience – that of 'shame-anxiety' (*uiat*), to which they mostly subject themselves (Beyer 2016).

We do not consider the invocation of shame an exclusively 'internalized' ideology, as it is through the outward expression of such an ideology that it becomes an element of interaction, of praxis, an act that is being performed by somebody and which is open to the interpretation of others.[18] Mortuary rituals in Kyrgyzstan in particular are built on moralizing public discourses and actions associated with shame-anxiety that lie exclusively in the domain of women, whereas men are expected to uphold and act according to Islamic law (Kyrg.: *shariat*). But during certain crucial life-cycle rituals, men depend on women to engage in practices, some of which violate *shariat*, to sustain important family relationships that can only be strengthened according to tradition (*salt boiuncha*). By carrying out elaborate exchange practices during mortuary rituals, women may transgress *shariat*, but they follow and uphold tradition (*salt*), according to which giving is a sign of respect – and to not give appropriately would trigger shame-anxiety, which turns out to be the graver concern.[19]

While Jarmila admits that the OBON work is not in and of itself deserving of respect (or even of her own self-respect), she nevertheless insists that her efforts to feed her children should command respect. This is more important to her than having work that is socially accepted. While she acknowledges that it was the economic incentive that brought her to the square in the first place, thus confirming the assumptions of administrators and even the public stereotype of OBON as demonstrators-for-hire, she also reflects critically on her behaviour and manages to turn a stigmatized practice into a morally worthy one. This reveals another aspect of traditionalization: actors strategically play expected types of behaviour against tolerated ones.

Kyrgyz stereotypes of woman as 'loud', 'gossipy' and 'emotional' do not operate exclusively in a negative way; they are enabling as well. While policing themselves and each other in terms of *uiat*, women are allowed (and in some cases expected) to display behaviour and perform tasks that would be considered inappropriate for men, particularly for aksakals. As with mortuary rituals, we see a gendered dimension in the public arena as two sides of the same political coin. In Kyrgyz politics, women lend further legitimacy to the performances of men in their roles as bearers of 'tradition' by displaying contrarian behaviour that challenges the decorum of tradition but reinforces cultural stereotypes. Male businessmen and politicians thus not only depend on aksakals to conjure up 'tradition', they also rely on women to help them carry out the unsavoury but crucial aspects of 'dirty politics' that get people removed from office or discredit political rivals. The behaviour that some women displayed during protests – screaming, cursing and even physically attacking protestors or police – was possible precisely because it could be rendered as 'typically female' behaviour. Also, it is culturally unacceptable to use force against women (at least in public), which allows women to act as a 'human shield' (Shabdanova 2012). This prohibition against touching or physically removing an unknown or older woman from public settings allowed OBON women to protest without direct sanctions. We argue that for the OBON women to perform according to this stereotype is just as related to Kyrgyz views of what is traditional as the aksakals' solemn speeches.

In general, OBON leaders were women who delegated tasks to other women – again similar to the exchange practices during mortuary rituals, where older women supervise their daughters and daughters-in-law as they act in the name of tradition, as Beyer (2016) has elaborated. But despite some women's active (if not institutionalized) leadership, OBON activities are masterminded by men. By staying in the background, these male patrons benefit from the capacities that female protest generates. It is here that we find a direct analogy to the aksakals. Taken together, these two categories of actors thus occupy diametrically opposed but complementary positions in political practice. They are both enabled by an understanding of tradition that, in the case of the aksakals, enshrines their 'wise' character as 'typical of an aksakal', and in the case of OBON – while lending itself to criticism of impropriety – at the same time legitimizes such behaviour as 'typical of women'. Women themselves invoke *uiat* to demonstrate their own self-awareness that their actions are not in line with a cultural model of tradition that does not endorse such public behaviour. Yet they are enabled by another aspect of that same model, as it labels their actions 'typically female'. We therefore argue that it is through rather than against *uiat* that OBON women are able to develop a political activist position which, to reiterate, has become necessary because of their vulnerable social and economic position in society.

Conclusion

Our investigation of political activism in Kyrgyzstan focused on aksakals and OBON women as two types of unusual political activists whose agency is differently enabled by invoking discourses and practices of tradition. Much of the literature on Central Asia has focused either on top-down processes of inventing tradition for the sake of the nation or on the weapons of the weak that counter these hegemonic tendencies. In contrast, we have shown that, when approached from a praxeological angle, some actors are able to tacitly exploit tradition's behavioural foundations and stereotypes, while others are constrained by the association of their behaviour with it. Male elders seek to realize their individual goals by performing within the publicly acknowledged realm of what is generally considered and respected as 'traditional' practice; OBON women, on the other hand, present themselves as economically and politically motivated actors but are seen by an observing local audience as engaging in 'shameful' practices. This portrayal, however, is in itself in line with a cultural model of acting according to tradition when it comes to public female performances, and is particularly striking when viewed as a counterpart to the performances of aksakals.

The invocation of tradition is not exclusively a top-down strategy, but gets employed in concrete situations by actors who know full well how to negotiate their behaviour in terms of others' expectations. While aksakals are acting out 'tradition' because they get to embody the positive aspects associated with it, OBON women end up performing their own negative clichés, even when trying to foreground political inclinations or economic needs. Their opinions on the nature and legitimacy of the protests thus remain divided. While some are satisfied with having achieved their personal aspirations and securing their livelihoods, others continue to defend their political activities in terms of citizenship duties and necessary opposition to state officials.

Our material demonstrates how, in the political arena in Kyrgyzstan, collective activities are not merely gendered, but interpreted through a traditionalist view of the intersection of gender and age. Factionalism, as displayed in the dynamics of 'meetings', *antimitings*, or the demonstrations of OBON, provides the background that allows elders to stage their 'aksakal-ness', which always demands appeals to harmony. But negative examples of anomic opposition facilitate the invocation of tradition as a perpetual demand, couched in culturally specific rhetoric and practices that are imposed on members of communities at various scales. Tradition is thus not just an instrument used by state institutions to enforce civic obedience, seen to be lacking in OBON activities, but finds more complex applications in practice, even among those who are accused of going against it.

Notes

1. See e.g. Gullette (2010); Reeves (2014); Laruelle and Engvall (2015); Doolotkeldieva (2015); Heathershaw and Cooley (2017); Ismailbekova (2017).
2. 'OBON' was coined in tongue-in-cheek analogy to OMON (Russ.: Otriad Militsii Osobogo Naznacheniia, Special Purpose Police Unit), an elite police force in Russia that is trained to fight organized crime and is also used to control demonstrations or mass protests. The B in OBON stands for *Bab*, which is itself short for *babushka* (grandma, old lady) and a slang word for women in general.
3. For research on elders' activism in other post-Soviet countries, see, e.g., Leipnik (2016) on the elderly in urban civic activism in Ukraine, and Edele (2008) on Soviet war veterans fighting for social benefits.
4. Kutmanaliev (2015) describes how, during the Osh riots in 2010, an Uzbek woman took leadership and coordinated defensive measures in a local Uzbek neighbourhood. While he notes that this was unusual, he describes the woman as having 'informal links with the local police' (470), being in charge of dealing with troublemakers in the neighbourhood (471), and having connections to the Kyrgyz community (472), thus acting well beyond the realm of her household.
5. The ethnonym 'Kyrgyz' itself is often attributed to the number 40, as is the image on the Kyrgyz flag, which depicts a sun with 40 rays, with a Kyrgyz *tündük* – the crisscrossed wooden structure at the peak of the roof of a yurt – in the centre.
6. The kalpak has also become a political statement in the music industry, with nationalist artists such as the Kyrgyz rapper Tata Ulan regularly wearing a kalpak in their music videos alongside other paraphernalia considered traditionally Kyrgyz.
7. For details see Erkebaeva (2017).
8. In 2005, the parliament of 120 deputies was entirely male. In 2015, still only 20% of the deputies were women, and this was after a gender quota had been introduced (UNDP Regional Human Development Report 2016).
9. For recent developments concerning 'heroism' in Kyrgyzstan, see Kojobekova (2014).
10. Megoran (2017, 85) cites one of the leaders who campaigned to have the female statue removed:

    > The reason is that in Kyrgyz culture, women never raise the *tündük*. That is done by the men. Women would do it on two occasions – if all the men were dead, or if all the men were away at war. There is an old curse, 'Your wife will hold the *tündük*', which means basically, I will kill you.'

11. Collective activities of elderly women that do exist – such as lamenting at funerals (*koshok* singing) – are not public in this sense.
12. See e.g., Kim et al. (2012), Shishkin (2013) and Szymanek (2012). For an overview of the public portrayal of OBON in local news and policy reports, see Alymkulova, Aitmatova, and Mamaraimov (2012).
13. See also Cleuziou's article in this special issue.
14. All personal names are pseudonyms.
15. Not all OBON are ethnic Kyrgyz, but most of the women Kojobekova interacted with were. For the purposes of this article, we are focusing on ethnic Kyrgyz women, but include this quote to

show that some of the discourses are shared among women across ethnic groups. Future research should address more explicitly the element of ethnic background and interethnic cooperation in women's political activism.

16. While speaking Kyrgyz throughout, the elders would use this Russian expression to indicate that they did not consider this particular way of speaking 'theirs' but as typical of a previous political era. See also Yurchak (2006).
17. In 2019, 500 *som* is the equivalent of about US$ 7.
18. This discussion draws on Beyer (2016) throughout.
19. See also the contributions by Cleuziou and Kudaibergenova in this special issue.

Acknowledgements

Data for this article were culled from Beyer's long-term ethnographic research between 2005 and 2015 in Talas Province in northern Kyrgyzstan and in the capital Bishkek, as well from interviews Kojobekova conducted throughout Kyrgyzstan over a period of several months in 2015. All names used in this article are pseudonyms. In Kojobekova's case we have also not specified places to protect the identity of her informants. The authors would like to thank Felix Girke, Juliette Cleuziou, Brian Donahoe and David Montgomery for helpful comments and suggestions.

Disclosure statement

No potential conflict of interest was reported by the authors.

Funding

This work was supported by the Cluster of Excellence "Cultural Foundations of Social Integration" at the University of Konstanz; the Max Planck Institute for Social Anthropology; and the Volkswagen Foundation.

References

Acosta, R. 2018. 'Toma-la ciudad': Intersubjective Activism in Guadalajara's Streets and City Museum. Accessed 7 January 2019. https://anthrosource.onlinelibrary.wiley.com/doi/full/10.1111/jlca.12386.

Alymkulova, A., J. Aitmatova, and A. Mamaraimov. 2012. "'OBON Kak Zerkalo': Razvitie Politicheskogo Aktivizma ili Ispol'zovanie Zhenskogo Resursa Dlya Tselei Grup Interesov v Kyrgyzstane. Tsentr Pomoshi Zhenshinam." Accessed 18 January 2018. http://wsc.kg/kg/obon-kak-zerkalo-razvitiepolitiche/ (site no longer active).

Attwood, L. 1999. *Creating the New Soviet Woman*. New York: St. Martens Press.

Beyer, J. 2005. "Die Aksakal-Gerichte in Kirgistan. Historische Entwicklung und aktuelle Situation einer traditionellen Rechtsinstanz in Zentralasien [The Aksakal Courts in Kyrgyzstan. Historical Development and Current Situation of a Traditional Legal Institution in Central Asia]." In *Rechtspluralismus in der islamischen Welt. Gewohnheitsrecht zwischen Staat und Gesellschaft*, edited by M. Kemper, and M. Reinkowski, 342–358. Berlin: De Gruyter.

Beyer, J. 2006. "Revitalisation, Invention and Continued Existence of the Kyrgyz Aksakal Courts: Listening to Pluralistic Accounts of History." *The Journal of Legal Pluralism and Unofficial Law* 38 (53–54): 141–176.

Beyer, J. 2010. "Authority as Accomplishment: Intergenerational Dynamics in Talas, Northern Kyrgyzstan." In *Eurasian Perspectives: In Search of Alternatives*, edited by A. Sengupta and S. Chatterjee, 78–92. New Delhi: Shipra.

Beyer, J. 2014a. "'There Is This Law' Performing the State in the Kyrgyz Courts of Elders." In *Ethnographies of the State in Central Asia: Performing Politics*, edited by M. Reeves, J. Rasanayagam, and J. Beyer, 99–123. Bloomington: Indiana University Press.

Beyer, J. 2014b. "Ordering Ideals: Accomplishing Well-Being in a Kyrgyz Cooperative of Elders." In *Negotiating Well-Being in Central Asia*, edited by D. Montgomery, 10–25. Abingdon and New York: Routledge.
Beyer, J. 2015. "Customizations of Law: Courts of Elders (*Aksakal* Courts) in Rural and Urban Kyrgyzstan." *Political and Legal Anthropology Review* 38 (1): 53–71.
Beyer, J. 2016. *The Force of Custom: Law and the Ordering of Everyday Life in Kyrgyzstan*. Pittsburgh: University of Pittsburgh Press.
Beyer, J., and F. Girke. 2015. "Practicing Harmony Ideology. Ethnographic Reflections on Community and Coercion." *Common Knowledge* 21 (2): 196–235.
Bichsel, C. 2009. *Conflict Transformation in Central Asia. Irrigation Disputes in the Ferghana Valley*. Abingdon, UK: Routledge.
Bridger, S. 1987. *Women in the Soviet Countryside*. Cambridge: Cambridge University Press.
Brusina, O. 2005. "Die Transformation der Adat-Gerichte bei den Nomanden Turkestans in der zweiten Hälfte des 19. Jahrhunderts [Transformation of Adat-Courts among the Nomads of Turkestan in the Second Half of the 19th Century]." In *Rechtspluralismus in der islamischen Welt: Gewohnheitsrecht zwischen Staat und Gesellschaft*, edited by M. Kemper and M. Reinkowski, 227–253. Berlin: De Gruyter.
Council of NGOs in Kyrgyzstan. 2014. "Alternative Report to the Fourth Periodic Report of the Kyrgyz Republic to the CEDAW Committee." Accessed 28 December 2017. http://wsc.kg/en/alternative-report-kyrgyzstan-2015/) (site no longer active).
Cummings, S., ed. 2010. *Domestic and International Perspectives on Kyrgyzstan's 'Tulip Revolution': Motives, Mobilizations and Meanings*. London: Routledge.
Cummings, S., and M. Ryabkov. 2008. "Situating the 'Tulip Revolution'." *Central Asian Survey* 27 (3-4): 241–252.
Doolotkeldieva, A. 2015. "Peripheral Protests as an Opportunity: 'Brokers' in Action." In *Kyrgyzstan Beyond 'Democracy Island' and 'Failing State'*, edited by M. Laruelle and J. Engvall, 59–79. Lanham: Lexington Books.
Edele, M. 2008. *Soviet Veterans of the Second World War: A Popular Movement in an Authoritarian Society, 1941–1991*. Oxford: Oxford University Press.
Edgar, A. 2004. *Tribal Nation: The Making of Soviet Turkmenistan*. Princeton: Princeton, University Press.
Engvall, J. 2015. "Why Are Public Offices Sold in Kyrgyzstan?" In *Kyrgyzstan Beyond 'Democracy Island' and 'Failing State'*, edited by M. Laruelle and J. Engvall, 39–59. Lanham: Lexington Books.
Erkebaeva, A. 2017. "Deputaty potrebovali nakazat' khoziaiku sobaki v kalpake." December 28. Accessed 10 March 2019. https://kloop.kg/blog/2017/12/28/deputaty-potrebovali-nakazat-hozyajku-sobaki-v-kalpake/.
Gullette, D. 2010. *The Genealogical Construction of the Kyrgyz Republic. Kinship, State and 'Tribalism'*. Kent: Global Oriental.
Hardtmann, E.-M. 2017. *South Asian Activists in the Global Justice Movement*. New Delhi: Oxford University Press.
Hasanov, R., S. Biybosunova, and S. Hasanova. 2009. "Assessing the Business Environment for Women's Entrepreneurship Development in the Kyrgyz Republic." Working Paper No. 3. International Labor Organization (ILO) Subregional Office for Eastern Europe and Central Asia. Accessed 10 March 2019. http://ilo.org/wcmsp5/groups/public/—europe/—ro-geneva/—sro-moscow/documents/publication/wcms_312485.pdf.
Heathershaw, J., and A. Cooley. 2017. *Dictators without Borders: Power and Money in Central Asia*. New Haven: Yale University Press.
Iskender, B. 2017. "Kak Reagirovat' na Shou o Kelinkakh Esli Vas ot Nego Toshnit?" Accessed 10 March 2019. https://kloop.kg/blog/2017/02/07/bektur-iskender-kak-reagirovat-na-shou-o-kelinkah-esli-vas-ot-nego-toshnit/.
Ismailbekova, A. 2016. "Constructing the Authority of Women through Custom: Bulak Village, Kyrgyzstan." *Nationalities Papers* 44 (2): 266–280.
Ismailbekova, A. 2017. *Blood Ties and the Native Son: Poetics of Patronage in Kyrgyzstan*. Bloomington: Indiana University Press.
Kandiyoti, D. 1988. "Bargaining with Patriarchy." *Gender and Society* 2 (3): 274–290.

Kandiyoti, D. 2007. "The Politics of Gender and the Soviet Paradox: Neither Colonized, Nor Modern?" *Central Asian Survey* 26 (4): 601–623.

Kim, A., A. Osmonalieva, I. Sikorskaya, and B. Rasulov. 2012. "Rent-a-Mob Protests in Central Asia: In Kyrgyzstan and Uzbekistan, Police and Politicians Recruit Women as Professional Campaigners or Just as Troublemakers." Accessed 10 March 2019. https://iwpr.net/global-voices/rent-mob-protests-central-asia.

Knyazev, A. 2005. *Gosudarstvenny Pereverot – 24 Marta 2005g. v. Kirgizii.* Bishkek: Obshchestvenny Fond Aleksandra Knyazeva.

Kocaoglu, T. 2009. "The Past as Prologue? Challenging the Myth of the Subordinate, Docile Woman in Muslim Central Eurasia." In *Gender Politics in Post-Communist Eurasia*, edited by L. Racioppi and K. O'Sullivan, 169–208. East Lansing: Michigan State University Press.

Kojobekova, A. 2014. "The Discourses of Romanticism and Heroism in the Post-Soviet Kyrgyzstan." *International Journal of Social Science and Humanity* 4 (5): 397–404.

Kutmanaliev, J. 2015. "Public and Communal Spaces and Their Relation to the Special Dynamics of Ethnic Riots: Violence and Non-Violence in the City of Osh." *International Journal of Sociology and Social Policy* 35 (7/8): 449–477.

Laruelle, M., and J. Engvall, eds. 2015. *Kyrgyzstan beyond 'Democracy Island' and 'Failing State': Social and Political Changes in a Post-Soviet Society.* Lanham: Lexington Books.

Leipnik, O. 2016. "The Elderly as a Force for Urban Civil Activism in Ukraine." In *Urban Grassroots Movements in Central and Eastern Europe*, edited by K. Jacobsson, 79–99. Farnham, Surrey: Ashgate.

Megoran, N. 2017. *Nationalism in Central Asia: A Biography of the Uzbekistan-Kyrgyzstan Boundary.* Pittsburgh, PA: University of Pittsburgh Press.

Meyer, J. W., and R. L. Jepperson. 2000. "The 'Actors' of Modern Society: The Cultural Construction of Social Agency." *Sociological Theory* 18 (1): 100–120.

Niiazova, M. 2015. "Kyrk Choro. Raskachat' Mezhnatsional'nuiu Lodku?" January 30. Accessed 10 March 2019. https://24.kg/obschestvo/6014_kyirk_choro_raskachat_mejnatsionalnuyu_lodku/.

Pelkmans, M. 2005. "On Transition and Revolution in Kyrgyzstan." *Focaal: Journal of Global and Historical Anthropology* 46: 147–157.

Reeves, M. 2014. *Border Work. Spatial Lives of the State in Rural Central Asia.* Ithaca and London: Cornell University Press.

Satybaldieva, E. 2018. "A Mob for Hire? Unpacking Older Women's Political Activism in Kyrgyzstan." *Central Asian Survey* 37 (2): 247–264.

Shabdanova, Asel'. 2012. "'Tret' Oproshennykh Priznali OBON Sposobnym Vliiat' na Reshenie Sotsial'nykh Problem." *Vechernyi Bishkek*, June 13. Accessed 10 March 2019. https://www.vb.kg/doc/191673_tret_oproshennyh_priznali_obon_sposobnym_vliiat_na_reshenie_socialnyh_problem.html.

Shishkin, P. 2013. *Restless Valley: Revolution, Murder, and Intrigue in the Heart of Central Asia.* New Haven, CT: Yale University Press.

Spector, R. 2017. *Order at the Bazaar: Power and Trade in Central Asia.* Ithaca, NY: Cornell University Press.

Suyarkulova, M. 2016. "Fashioning the Nation: Gender and Politics of Dress in Contemporary Kyrgyzstan." *Nationalities Papers* 44 (2): 247–265.

Szymanek, M. 2012. "OBON: Rent-A-Mob Groups in the Volatile Kyrgyzstani Reality." December 6. Accessed 10 March 2019. http://neweasterneurope.eu/2012/12/06/obon-rent-a-mob-groups-in-the-volatile-kyrgyzstani-reality-2/.

Temirkulov, A. 2010. "Informal Actors and Institutions in Mobilization: The Periphery in the 'Tulip Revolution'." In *Domestic and International Perspectives on Kyrgyzstan's 'Tulip Revolution: Motives, Mobilizations and Meanings'*, edited by S. Cummings, 93–110. London: Routledge.

UNDP Regional Human Development Report. 2016. "Case Study on Combating Gender Inequality on Political Participation in Kyrgyzstan." Accessed 10 March 2019. http://www.kg.undp.org/content/dam/kyrgyzstan/Publications/gender/Case%20study_Eng10Oct2016.pdf.

Yurchak, A. 2006. *Everything Was Forever Until It Was No More. The Last Soviet Generation.* Princeton, NJ: Princeton University Press.

Traditionalization, or the making of a reputation: women, weddings and expenditure in Tajikistan

Juliette Cleuziou

ABSTRACT
This article aims to show how traditionalization is enforced by women in Tajikistan in the realm of marriage, focusing on the economic dimension of life cycle rituals: ritual expenditure and gift-giving. It shows that from women's points of view, performing ceremonial competition may itself be a resource to recover their reputation, for example when a matrimonial rupture has harmed it. Focusing on single mothers, it demonstrates how practices of traditionalization performed by women can be directed at addressing gender constraints and stereotypes, such as the normative relation between marriage and femininity, and how they may also secure women's separate sphere of competence and relative financial autonomy.

Introduction

Tajikistan, like the other post-Soviet Central Asian republics, has been witnessing a form of neotraditionalism at the political level. The government ruled by Emomali Rahmon has been elaborating a revivalist discourse on 'tradition' (*an'ana*) which aims to build political legitimacy by shaping historical memory and social relations (Adams 2010; Direnberger 2014; Hughes 2017; Lemon 2013; Nourzhanov 2001; Thibault 2013; see also Beyer and Finke in the introduction to this special issue). Invoking 'tradition' and references to historical heroic ancestors have been widely used by governments to assert and legitimize their authority, producing a well-established narrative on the need for Central Asian republics to recover their traditional way of life after the Soviet interlude.

Gender norms and relations in particular have been a central object of attention and discussion, a concern that these nationalist projects share with other nationalisms in the world (Yuval-Davis 1993) as well as with the former Soviet regime (Cleuziou and Direnberger 2016; Direnberger 2014; Harris 2004; Kamp 2006). However, as Kandiyoti (2007) argued a decade ago, framing people's current practices through the binary prism of Soviet modernity and nationalist (re)traditionalism is misleading, as conceptions and practices of what is locally considered modern (*zamonavi*, also often translated by the Russian term *sovremennyj*) or traditional (*an'anavi*) are very much intertwined – a consideration that my article will illustrate through the example of Tajikistan. Not only did the Soviet period allow a great part of customary and religious practices to cohabit with the claimed modernity of Soviet ideology; the current post-independence Tajik regime that glorifies national traditions also has to face an unprecedented diversification in modes of life, family patterns and gendered divisions of labour entailed by post-war rapid urbanization and male out-migration.

In this article, rather than trying to identify or separate what is tradition from what it is not (as neotraditionalism tries to), I focus on practices that people label 'traditional', recognizing them to be a source of authority to organize practices, concomitantly with an endeavour to perpetuate or reproduce them. In particular, I investigate practices referred to as 'traditional' that prevail among Tajik women by focusing on the performance of wedding ceremonies and marriage payments. In this female-dominated realm of action, Tajik women try to show their ability to mobilize networks of acquaintances and produce a sense of lavishness to impress their neighbours and sustain their good reputation.

This article is situated in a context where marriage practices, an unavoidable dimension of normative femininity, have been brutally disrupted since the collapse of the Soviet Union. The civil war (1992–1997), followed by waves of male migration to Russia, brought about a considerable increase in divorces, separations, wife abandonment and widowhood, leaving women without the social protection that marital unions supposedly offer them.[1] While marriage and relations to in-laws have remained central to women's sociality and security in Tajikistan, these (often tragic) events lead them to imagine alternative coping strategies. In the end, many women find themselves in a situation of matrimonial abnormality, which might be experienced as a failing or deficiency.

Recent work on Central Asia has regularly addressed the intersection of tradition and gender, with a focus on women. Werner (2009) showed for example how narratives on tradition and shame have reframed and reinforced patriarchal ideology in post-Soviet Kazakhstan, especially regarding women's decision in marriage. Commercio (2015, p. 2) argued that young women in urban settings in Kyrgyzstan and Tajikistan tend to sympathize with a certain idea of retraditionalization, defined as 'a return to traditional values, family life, [and] religion, including women being moved out of the workforce', although the extent to which these narratives affect women's lives remains to be explored. Roche (2016) demonstrated that traditional practices linked to social and biological reproduction and control over women's bodies have been replaced by a medicalized approach during the Soviet period and since independence. She highlights how this medical approach perpetuates traditional views on women's roles as spouses and mothers, a consideration that consistently serves the nationalist project.[2] More broadly, research on tradition and gender has shown how tradition reinforces patriarchal ideology and restrictions on women's behaviour and mobility. This work has yielded important empirical and theoretical insights into the reproduction of patriarchal relations. Less attention has been paid to the spaces of women's agency in this specific constraining context (though see Cleuziou 2016; Roche 2015). The current article contributes to this emergent literature by showing how women can use 'tradition' to restore their reputation and feed social positioning, or even upward social mobility.

Drawing from the case of Madina, a single mother who celebrated her daughter's wedding in 2013 in Dushanbe, I will show how she strives to organize lavish ceremonies, to orchestrate them in a 'traditional' manner, to reverse the stigma of shame associated with her matrimonial marginality. In doing so, I seek to explore forms of traditionalization 'from the bottom' (Fathi 2004). Traditionalization is understood not as a return to past practices but as a performance where people, ideas, values and norms interact at a given moment, according to a certain order, and are collectively acknowledged as valuable and 'traditional' (see also the introduction to this special issue by Beyer and Finke). Although one case does not suffice for a statement of general features in a country as diverse as Tajikistan, it enables us to understand how negotiating traditional practices such as marriage ceremonies may be empowering for single women, and how tradition, gender and shame intersect with women's agency in a constraining environment.

I proceed by presenting the collective dynamics of wedding organization illustrated by Madina's daughter's marriage, and how the marriage offers stages for practices of traditionalization. I then explore how 'the traditional' may be changing, based on the example of marriage payments. I conclude by showing how traditionalization connects to issues of prestige and reputation, and that it may be used as a tool for single women such as Madina to restore their reputation or prevent the fear of losing it.

Organizing wedding ceremonies

Madina's daughter, Samina, got married in June 2013. I was closely involved in the wedding organization since I was one of the bride's witnesses (*yanga*, lit. 'uncle's wife' or 'brother's wife', and more broadly any older women related by marriage), who would accompany her during her first night at her in-laws' house. Madina is a widow who raised her three children (by two different fathers) by herself. She used to be a nurse but now sells food and runs a guesthouse for tourists in Dushanbe. When Madina agreed to marry her elder daughter off, she undertook huge expenses to celebrate the wedding in the most lavish manner, even though she was the only working person in the household. While putting herself into debt, she also put Samina in a delicate situation, since she was only 17 at the time, too young to legally marry. Yet, doing otherwise, Madina feared, would have led people to gossip (*gaybat kardan*): she lives without a husband, and Samina without a father, a situation sometimes referred to by the pejorative expression *be sohib*, 'without a master'. Madina had already received several marriage proposals for her daughter, and she decided to accept the last one so as to avoid any doubts concerning Samina's honour, and broadly for her reputation (*nomus*, in Tajik, may be used for both meanings but is particularly applied to women[3]). Madina gathered close to USD10,000 to spend on her daughter's wedding, most of which was used for the celebration itself (*tuy-i duxtar*, lit. 'daughter's wedding') and to compile a considerable dowry (*ruzgor, mol*) of manufactured goods (furniture, jewellery, dresses, cosmetics, cushions and mattresses, bed and linen, etc.), which was later transferred to Samina's husband's house.

Here, I would like to highlight two important dimensions of Tajik weddings, which are found across the great variety of wedding ceremonies that exist in the country. First, during the ceremony and at each step of concluding the marriage – there are often over 15 such steps, including those before and after the wedding day per se (Abashin 2015; Cleuziou 2016; Kisliakov 1959; Roche 2014; Sukhareva 1940; Tett 1996) – Madina was constantly surrounded by other women: her two sisters, her sisters-in-law, her nieces, her neighbours, her friends and me. A week before the wedding, those who did not live nearby arrived to stay at Madina's house; all of them helped in preparing the food and decorating the rooms where the guests would be hosted. One morning, on entering one of the rooms, I saw that Madina's relatives were assembling small packages of gifts, filled with textiles, sweets, headscarves, shampoos, soaps and combs, to redistribute to Samina's in-laws during the ceremony. This moment is very sensitive because women are deciding how to distribute the gifts to their future in-laws, which will then publicly mark and acknowledge social positions according to family, gender and generation relations.[4] Samina's mother-in-law should receive more than her aunt-in-law, but what about her sister-in-law? The procedure gives rise to endless conversations about textile quality, the glamorous style of the groom's sisters, the conservative tone of his grandmother, and the modern style of his parents. Every member of the groom's family is 'evaluated' to be sure that he or she will receive gifts according to their position, but also according to the impacts on their own image (being religious, modern, generous, having taste, etc.). As such, decisions require the participation of trustworthy people. Although in this specific case the word 'tradition' itself is not pronounced, the reproduction of practices considered right and necessary is at stake. In this particular moment, women draw on tradition as a cultural model: that is, as a way to legitimize their actions to prescribe forms of collaboration and mutual help among kin and close neighbours; but the aim is also to impress and compete by means of wealthy gifts made to the future in-laws and to neighbours.

Another moment during Samina's wedding is significant: when she arrived at her husband's house, she would have to go through different rites of integration into the house, from being unveiled (*ruy binon*) and kissed by her husband's female kin, to kneading bread dough (*sari sulfa*) and hiding behind a cloth during the first night. However, Samina's mother-in-law asked several times: 'How should it be done?' Should the bride knead the bread first, and then look at herself in the mirror? Should a young boy, picked from among the guests, unveil the bride with a stick, or should the mother-in-law do it? How should the gifts be offered to the bride? Are women supposed to dance for the bride before or after kissing her? Such discussions, which typically take place in the kitchen with kin, friends and neighbours, are quite frequent during ceremonies and show that the 'rules' of tradition need to be debated in light of a concrete situation among the people present, including, most importantly, the guests. Thus, one can say that the wedding is a performance where the audience become active participants and the order of ritual details are worked out collectively, at least to a certain extent. Yet, most women actually know how to accomplish the rituals: the point is rarely about knowledge. Some rituals are known to be unavoidable, such as the religious ceremony itself (*nikoh*) or the transfer of the bride to her in-laws' house. Others can be negotiated: unveiling and dancing, for example. But what is at stake for the main organizers is to gain collective approval – a point I will develop later on. For now, it is worth noting that the purpose of these discussions is rather to show the host's will to pull together, in order to receive sufficient approval of how the ceremonies are being enacted. This shows how women collectively reproduce, negotiate and alter the rules of traditional marriage performance, reinforcing their own experience and authority in the realm of ceremonies. It also demonstrates the importance women seem to put in performing – even *staging* – relations of reciprocity during these festive events. Such collaboration is not only about doing but also about 'showing doing' (Schechner 2013). Tajik weddings are indeed not only about showing wealth and networks, they are also stages on which to display an (often ephemeral) wealth, such as in Madina's case, and an occasion to receive acknowledgment of one's behaviour as 'traditional' and thereby in line with the expectations of others.

Staging traditions

Analysing narratives of 'tradition' among the Choctaw in North America, Mould (2005, 268) argues that 'only when speakers construct contexts communally recognized as referencing the traditional can the process be labelled *traditionalization*'. This search for collective approval and proper performance during weddings constitutes such a moment, when participants construct 'the traditional' and negotiate how new or modern aspects, such as certain goods, clothing and practices, may be integrated. The habits of toasting and drinking alcohol, for example, which derive from Russian Soviet practices, or the more recent trend of avoiding any kind of alcoholic drinks, indicate how 'tradition' always needs to be investigated at a particular historical and social moment. While drinking was once 'traditional' during weddings (including toasting), now not-drinking has become standard practice and is advocated as 'traditionally Tajik'. As Stephan-Emmrich has argued, the latter process results from the combination of several phenomena: the growing interest in Islamic practices, which serve as a coping strategy in an uncertain socio-economic environment, as well as the desire to partake in a worldwide Islamic modernity and its related consumption practices (Stephan 2010; Stephan-Emmrich and Mirzoev 2016; see also McBrien 2009). Other examples include renting a bride's white wedding dress (in contrast with the black dress, covering the whole body, that women used to sew at the beginning of the twentieth century), going for a romantic walk in botanic gardens and filming the event on a DVD, or buying bedding furniture as part of the dowry. Such practices reflect not only the evolution of consumption in the twentieth century but also how objects and practices travel in and out of 'tradition'.

In organizing her daughter's impressive wedding, Madina subjected herself to the expectations of others (see also Beyer 2016, 145ff.) in terms of what one should do when marrying off one's child: being able to gather and redistribute wealth, food and entertainment in a short time, and to the benefit of her guests. A wedding is a 'total event' (*fait social total* in the Maussian sense) consisting of economic, social and ritual components, between which 'it would be futile to attempt distinctions … since the participants themselves experience these as a seamless totality' (Kandiyoti and Azimova 2004, 336). This skilful demonstration of upholding 'tradition' through wedding performances will later be transformed, via further gift-exchange and gossip, into prestige, enforcing Madina's reputation as an honourable woman who does things properly (*zani bo farhang/madaniyat,* literally 'a woman with culture').

Performing one's status is a consistent part of building 'the communal' (Kandiyoti and Azimova 2004). Although the word 'tradition' itself is not mentioned, I would argue that such moments are 'conscious and explicit efforts at traditionalization' (Mould 2005, 257), which create and reproduce specific assumptions about those practices that should be enacted. There is some flexibility in this search for collective approval, which, in the end, has to come to an agreement on what should be done. Given the scheme of collaboration and collective discussion that characterizes wedding performances, it is no surprise that a wedding becomes an example to follow – or to surpass – the next time, constructing a cultural model of ritual performances.

Thus, practices of traditionalization in Tajik matrimonial life occur during collective performances, which imply a form of reciprocity and of collective approval that allows the model to be applied to other situations. Such efforts at emulation have led, in recent years, to a remarkable inflation of expenditure, which tends to create more obstacles for certain sections of the population, who are not as rich or who do not have access to resources.

Changing the 'traditional': when bride price returns as dowry

To illustrate how the 'traditional' has been changing in Tajikistan, I focus now on recent transformations of marriage payments, where the 'traditional' bride-price, given by the groom's parents to that of the bride, has become secondary, ousted by the 'newly traditional' practice of dowry transfer, which consists of gifts the bride receives from her parents and brings to her in-laws' house. According to my informants, from Dushanbe and the mountainous areas of Darvoz, dowry transfer seems to have developed in the late 1960 and the 1970s, when Central Asia was living prosperously under the Soviet regime (a period described as 'mature socialism' by Koroteyeva and Makarova 1998), but really accelerated in the 1980s, and then again after the interruption of the civil war (1992–1997), under the influence of remittances sent by migrants from Russia.[5]

The rise of ceremonial expenditure has been underlined in research on the region during both the Soviet and the post-Soviet periods (Koroteyeva and Makarova 1998; Pétric 2004; Poliakov 1992). However, rare are the observers who have also underlined the changing patterns of marriage payments (though see Reeves 2012). Abashin (1999) suggested that the boundaries between the different types of marriage payments in Central Asia should be taken as relatively fluid. If the terminology that includes designation of bride price[6], dowry[7] or *mahr*[8] is rooted in specific historical processes, the practical boundaries between these objects are difficult to draw because of the overwhelming number of reciprocal gift exchanges in ceremonial contexts. My own data also show that the distinction between bride price, dowry and *mahr* is not always easy to see, even for the people invloved. Yet, a general statement has been circulating in Tajikistan in the past decades: parents have been paying more for their daughter's weddings than before, exceeding what is usually spent for their sons'. No one I talked to seemed to have an explanation for this phenomenon, yet many agreed that 'our grandmothers used to get married with a pair of golden earrings and a pillow, and that was it'. But marriage payments have been changing, and bride-price apparently does not represent the main transfer as it used to be. Many people emphasized that dowry expenses have increased, especially in recent years. Marrying off a daughter now often appears more expensive than marrying off a son, because, as one woman from Qarotegin put it, 'When you marry off your son, everything comes back with the bride, and even more!'

But when marrying off one's daughter, one loses the bride and the dowry. Now, the dowry includes the transformation of the bride-price money and cotton into material goods, which will move with the bride to her in-laws' house. Yet, expectations for dowries have been significantly exceeding the sum given in the bride-price in the first place, because today a typical dowry includes, in addition to the usual bride's clothing (*sar-u po*, literally 'head and foot') and personal items (such as gold jewellery), a full set of kitchen appliances, including a microwave, refrigerator and mixer, sometimes an oven, and all the vessels in different shapes and colours. It also includes bed furniture, such as a Western type of bed, a dressing table and a cupboard, in complement to traditional mattresses and blankets. To this can be added a television, carpets or a sofa, according to people's means, as well as all the gifts made to the in-laws in the course of the various (and often numerous) ceremonies. Along with the dowry itself, ceremonies where these items are displayed (*tuqquz binon*, 'seeing the dowry', or *choy gashtak*, 'gathering for tea') have been developing. This has led to the point where families in many different parts of the country[9] now often organize a 'daughter's/bride's wedding' (*tuy-i dukhtar/arus*), as Madina did for her daughter, before the 'son's/groom's wedding' (*tuy-i bacha/domod*) – the latter usually being considered the wedding proper.

As mentioned by Abashin, both types of transfers, from the groom's and from the bride's sides, entail cycles of gift-giving and mutual indebtedness. Yet, the reversal of marriage's main financial roles from bride price to dowry – a process that has also been observed in other parts of the world[10] – shows the growing importance of conspicuous consumption in staging prestige and family status.[11] The flows of money sent by migrants from Russia (remittances), the Chinese production of manufactured goods, and the lack of alternative spheres of investment (in a country where racketing and corruption prevent small businesses from flourishing) seem to have put ceremonial expenditures at the centre of reputation and prestige display.[12] Moreover, wedding ceremonies that alternate between the groom and the bride's house terminate, after the wedding celebration per se, with transfers from the bride's side to the groom's side.[13] At these different occasions, dowry transfers are repeatedly operated but rarely entail negotiations between families or any expectation of 'counter gift'. In the context where weddings follow an inflationary process, final ceremonies tend to be even more expensive, which could explain the parents' consideration for their daughters' weddings.

The spread of dowry transfer, as a 'traditional' practice characterized by the exponential cost of marrying one's daughter, does not occur without a paradox: the circulation of goods it entails also circulates representations of modern consumption, materialized by specific goods such as household appliances or furniture. More generally, the increasing role of financial means to demonstrate status and power has led to the development of dowry as a social marker of family prestige that also plays out with images of the modern way of life. Dowry transfers have become a 'traditional' way of concluding a marriage, yet the traditional here does not rely on a justification such as 'doing as our forefathers did' but rather on what the neighbours are actually doing.

Finally, the dowry offers the possibility of claiming tradition through reinvented ceremonies and money transfers. In fact, the accumulation and distribution of the dowry are also based on women's collaboration and competition. The dowry has generalized inside the matrimonial system because it fits in the general frame of weddings in the country that the description of Madina's celebration aimed to illustrate: on the one hand, collaboration and redistribution among kin and neighbours to accumulate and distribute; and on the other, lavishness and competition for social status between the families getting married. The dowry seems to have been traditionalized because it proceeds from social relations structured by reputational mechanisms, as I explore in more detail below.

Gaining and preserving one's reputation

Traditionalization thus consists in the performance of specific practices that allow one to garner collective approval and maintain one's position in the group and all the different networks involved in daily life. As Mould (2005, 289) puts it,

> Traditionalizing moves are often used to establish authority and authenticity for the individual in the act of performance. In this way, the traditional becomes more than an idea: it is a resource actively manipulated for specific and often personal ends.

Performing tradition to gain collective approval is, indeed, a resource in Tajikistan. Why is it so? I argue that ceremonial expenditures convey a moral stand of respectability that feeds one's reputation when they are accomplished according to the others' expectations, that is, according to 'the traditional'. Far from opposing emotions and money, or moral standards and personal interests (Zelizer 2000), wedding ceremonies in Tajikistan conflate practices of competition and mutual help, of expectation and support between the hosts and their guests. The connection between conspicuous spending and social status in Central Asia is now well acknowledged (Nalivkin and Nalivkina 1886; Poliakov 1992; Koroteyeva and Makarova 1998; Abashin 2009; Danzer et al. 2013). I would like now to insist on the moral dimension of this spending, as the case of Madina shows well how wealth, distributed under the seal of traditional ceremonies, is thought to influence one's reputation.

When I asked Madina why she would spend so much money that she did not have (close to USD10,000) on her daughter's wedding, she answered, 'So that nobody can say to my daughter that she grew up without a father.' Hospitality and prodigality, especially in marriage celebrations, are expected to work as compensation for the lack of a husband in the family. Her daughter's wedding ceremony should contribute to securing and strengthening her and her daughter's reputation. She sought to impress others and to gain their collective approval. Among all the women I met, this aspect was emphasized: celebrating lavishly can act as proof of one's morality and the respectability of one's family (*nomus dorad,* 's/he/it has honour', 's/he/it is respectable'). Here, I should mention that in families where both parents take part in the organization of the wedding, the father's role is crucial in both agreeing on the spouse and in financing the ceremonies. In families where women head the household, reputation, and its moral connotation derived from conspicuous spending, takes greater significance. Madina is a widow (*beva*), along with many others, due to the civil war, I which so many men lost their lives. Within this group are also repudiated and divorced women, whose number has risen since the 2000s, when men began seeking work in Russia. The single women's life stories I collected show a constant concern to distance themselves from possible accusations of being playgirls or prostitutes.[14]

In the context where conforming to tradition allows women to confirm their status and maintain their reputation, it becomes clear that traditionalization is a process through which women may prevent such humiliating accusations as well as securing specific resources and sociability inside their networks of acquaintances. In Tajikistan, inviting many guests make possible multiple future exchanges, among them the gifts of basins full of food products, sweets and textiles that women traditionally offer one another. Thus, their own marriage and, later, their children's marriage – and especially their son's – are important steps in building their social capital. Single women such as Madina show their ability to circulate wealth, redistribute goods and celebrate marriage *as if* they were married, by taking on the roles of both mother and father (Cleuziou 2017). More generally, conforming to tradition by holding celebrations and adhering to gift-exchange practices, as well as enforcing gender norms such as women's modesty, marriage and motherhood, are the most secure ways to protect one's reputation. Performing tradition and performing expected gender roles are different but complementary facets of constructing one's reputation in the context of patriarchal ideology.

What is reputation about?

A driving force in these festive performances is, as Madina shows, reputation. In Tajikistan, reputation (*nomus, obru*) is closely linked to the fear of losing it and being afflicted by shame (*ayb, sharm*). Male and female reputation can be generated by family position, professional status, political power, religious knowledge, wealth and appropriate behaviour, all domains linked to specific resources – for which men and women both compete, but usually in distinct domains. The expressions *be nomus* and *be obru* ('without honour' and 'without virtue') are used to describe both men's and women's misbehaviour. They are synonyms of another word, *sharm*, which is widely used in Tajik when commenting on behaviour, and in particular women's behaviour. The expression '*sharmanda!*' may be uttered in a variety of situations and about a variety of behaviours, going from modesty to disgrace. It can be addressed to a misbehaving child, or to adult women who are said to be seen in an improper or even indecent situation (e.g., 'she was talking late at night to an unknown man'). In the latter case, the word appears quite offensive and should be taken as such. It could be translated as 'shameful' in its strongest meaning. In this dimension, it partially covers the meaning of the Kyrgyz word *uiat*. Analysing mourning rituals in Kyrgyzstan, Beyer (2016) shows that people – and women in particular – feel compelled to participate in gift-exchanges despite their onerous costs and that they explain their behaviour in the name of *uiat*. In this context, *uiat* should be understood as preventive shame-anxiety that is being generated when anticipating a conduct that others may judge negatively, and thus should be avoided.[15] It implies that what the others think matters greatly in the way one reflects one's own behaviour and conduct: 'It is self-reflection and self-evaluation of individuals more than external sanctioning by others that leads to the performance judged to be 'according to *salt*' [custom]' (Beyer 2016, 148–149). In the situations I observed in Tajikistan, *sharmanda* may be a preventive emotion, in that it is also often used to comment negatively on someone's behaviour, in particular during moments of gossiping, which would often take the following pattern. A woman would tell a story of another's misbehaviour, and her audience would go '*tttt sharmanda!*' – enacting the moral condemnation of improper conduct and hence reasserting the norms of the group (on the normative and performative aspect of gossip, see Abrahams 1970).[16] Thus, the term seems to be used both in preventive and sanctioning ways, even if it takes the form of indirect comments.

Whether in lavish ceremonies or in gossip, people do take into account the potential consequences in the eyes of their relatives, neighbours, friends and colleagues before acting, but they are also keen on sanctioning others' immorality and misconduct. As the philosopher Claudia Origgi (2015, 97) argues, people face the problem of how to evaluate one another's reputations: the reliability of the 'signal' on which reputation is built is a central matter to all in the community. She gives as an example the signal 'studied/worked in Oxford University': it seems a robust one for evaluating one's reputation, especially in the academic sphere. Yet, when Gatsby, Fitzgerald's eponymous character, says that he studied in Oxford, people from the elite do not perceive the sign as coherent with his behaviour. Reputation in fact is not built only from social positioning and objective signals (such as 'Oxford') but also from the perception that people have of this positioning. This is why reputation is a 'meta-representation' (71): it is the opinion that one draws from others' opinions, the representation of a representation, that indicates what one should think of others but always remains subject to change.

In the context of Tajikistan, I argue that performing tradition (through wedding celebrations, for example) acts an emic signal for building one's reputation but which is always grounded in uncertainty. Madina's strategic positioning 'in accordance with tradition' may be interpreted in different ways by her surroundings. This explains the need for collective approval that she strives to earn through her daughter's wedding. Being part of a group implies a part of respect towards (even deference to) the social authority of the group itself, its norms and rules. However, as reputation is never won once and for all, it 'constantly creates uncertainties and generates anxieties of social positioning which do not seem to be ascertainable' (Origgi 2015, 114, my translation). The part of uncertainty is the source of anxiety that Beyer named 'shame anxiety'. Establishing a map of people's positioning in the social world according to their reputation is impossible because reputation is never objective nor objectively defined in diachronic terms. One can understand Madina's endeavours to remain part of the group by conforming to the ceremonial game – like the Kyrgyz protagonists of the funerals described by Beyer (2016, 135–154), who may also indebt themselves to perform what they understand as unavoidable. Not only is it a way to maintain harmony (*yntymak*) in the Kyrgyz context; it is also a way to maintain access to the 'group' (as vague as this definition can be) and to networks of information and services, as well as to preserve a certain sense of security and belonging. Beyer's (2016, 154) interlocutors say they are 'destroying money' by spending their savings on gifts during funerals, but they still feel compelled to do it to remain inside the 'communal' (Kandiyoti and Azimova 2004). My own informants were saying approximately the same and would also often complain about ceremonial costs – but still performing them, as they think they are expected to, in a context where community matters. Even though the law in Tajikistan has made such spending illegal, ways to bypass the legislation remain numerous – an aspect that will be explored in the final part of this article.

Regulating tradition, preventing traditionalization?

Though many of my informants said that they agree with President Rahmon's efforts to limit them, they continue spending huge amounts of money on ceremonies. Indeed, just as in Uzbekistan, the Tajik government has been trying to regulate the inflation of wedding expenses. A law was passed on 7 June 2007, locally referred to as Tanzim (regulation).[17] It aims to regulate 'the development of society, tradition and celebration, and preserve values of authentic national culture and respect for people's traditions, to raise the socio-economic level of life.'[18] However, since 2007, only a few cases of fines have been reported in the media (e.g., Najibullah and Salimov 2015), and most people continue with lavish banquets. And various strategies have been implemented to bypass the law, such as transferring the dowry at night, or organizing several ceremonies on different days and with different guests. Mukhabbat, a Dushanbe dweller in her forties, once explained to me that

> Sometimes poor people want to act like rich people so as not to feel poor in front of others, and spend a lot of money.... I agree with the law that our president has passed. Obviously if my neighbour organizes a big wedding, I would like to do the same, and I would like my son to be rich, too. But on the other side, I am happy that the president wrote this law so that I do not have to do it, because I cannot. It allows everyone to stand at the same level. What is the point in organizing such fat weddings and losing all your money this way? You can do it in an 'average' way, so that the parents can also live a normal life [afterwards]. If today you lose everything when organizing a wedding, where will you find your food tomorrow? Are you going to indebt yourself even more?

Still, Mukhabbat concluded our meeting by saying, 'Of course, I would like my daughter to celebrate a rich wedding.'

Marriage expenses are one way to study the discrepancy between what people generally say, what they say they do, and what they actually do (Reeves 2012; Beyer 2016, 18). While many people agree with the law, they cannot imagine constraining their own marriage accordingly (the obvious example being that of the president himself, when he lavishly celebrated his son's wedding in 2009).

The 2007 law identifies three forms of ceremonies whose conditions of celebration are restricted (*an'ana* [tradition], *dzhashn* [celebration], and *marosim* [ceremony] – the law gives detailed lists for each category), mentioning for example the number of guests (no more than 150 for a wedding), the type of relations to the guests (family and others), the quantity and the type of food (e.g., the amount of rice one can cook), and the timing (three-hour ceremonies during weekends only), as well as sanctions in case of transgression. Yet, many other 'details' usually escape control. In particular, the spending on gifts and food, and the number of actual gatherings organized usually go far beyond the spirit of the law.

Ten years later (11 August 2017), an amendment to the law reinforced state control and forbade all 'excessive' (tj. *izrofkori va ziedaravi*) celebrations, such as for Ramazon, Idi Qurbon or circumcision feasts (the latter may be organized at the hospital only, until the 21st day after birth).[19] Nowadays, people seem more aware of the legislation, and more have been fined by local authorities or the police. There is now a chance that the inflationary process will be slowed, but only the coming years will show.[20]

In addition to the state's goals of framing wedding ceremonies with nationalist ambitions and to the slow spreading of frugal ceremonies in the name of Islam, another socio-economic factor impacts greatly on ceremonial spending (Trevisani 2016). Access to cheap goods from China, Turkey or Russia tends in many ways to standardize ceremonial expenditures, but the fact that many Tajik men go to Russia as labour migrants, often for several years, has visible consequences for matrimonial life. Indeed, Samina's marriage, like many others, did not last long, barely a year and a half. Her husband divorced her ('taloq'), which is an illustration of the current trend, both a consequence of transnational life in families and of the tensions between individual desires and family expectations. She could get part of her dowry back, but only part – and she was lucky to get anything, since it is far from being a general rule. Despite being aware of this, women like Madina still feel compelled to celebrate lavishly, as if there was no alternative (such as a modest celebration), which shows that expensive dowries have less to do with concluding long-lasting marriage relations (although people do hope that the marriage will last) than with the issue of reputation. Madina's case is not unique in Dushanbe, nor in the rest of the country.

One has to remember that earning money, in Tajik society, usually means that one has an obligation to redistribute: wealth should circulate. And what would be the alternative to these expenses, anyway? In a country where starting a business always includes a very high risk of being robbed or racketed, and where trust in institutions mostly depends on patronage and personal networks, how could investing in social relations hurt? Performing ceremonies and building one's reputation under the seal of tradition remains a relatively secure investment, compared to unsecure investments in businesses, for example. It is interesting, however, that people's own justifications do not emphasize rationality but reputation, emotion and the fear of being accused of not acting properly.

Conclusion: Traditionalization as a resource for building women's reputation

Throughout this article, I have elaborated on the idea that traditionalization is a conscious practice aimed at reproducing what should be done, and thus at preventing shaming and protecting one's reputation. Rather than referring to a common past, traditionalization takes place in a context where community matters for one's social positioning, which is mediated through the building up of one's reputation. Traditionalization appears as an endeavour to portray one's behaviour as in line with 'what has always been done', and as such, affirm one's reputation. By performing ceremonies in a 'traditional' way, and 'showing doing' (Schechner 2013) by earning collective approval, Madina publicly demonstrates her group identity, which allows her to remain part of a group from which her matrimonial situation (as a single mother) may have marginalized her. Through the marriage ceremonies, Madina implicitly argues that though she is not married, she is respectable *as if* she were; she thus addresses gender constraints and stereotypes, such as the normative relation between femininity, reputation and marriage. Her case also shows that practices of traditionalization may secure women's separated sphere of activities and relative financial autonomy: Madina is able to gather money for the ceremony thanks to her own networks. In doing so, Madina bargains her participation to the reproduction of women's 'demarcated sphere of competence' (Beyer 2016, 177), which may be enabling,[21] rather than one of simple compliance with a patriarchal bargain (Kandiyoti 1988). If practices of traditionalization tend to reproduce gender constraints, and especially the close links between marriage and acceptable femininity, they also offer 'solutions' to women such as Madina who do not match gender normativity in the realm of economic exchange and ritual celebration Circulating wealth may overcome gender anomy, and honouring one's relations may silence, at least temporarily, gender norms. What Madina's story highlights are the tensions of simultaneous phenomena that cut across Tajik society: on the one hand, the tension between the increasing role of prestige and money (and spending) as social markers and the remaining importance of community relations (through reputational mechanisms), and on the other hand, the discrepancy between normative gender roles and actual economic issues that have led women to take over roles usually occupied by men.

Interestingly, this cultural model women draw on is not justified by a legacy of the past: they refer less to what their forefathers (supposedly) did than to what their neighbours actually did (last week, last month, last year). In this perspective, reproducing traditional practices is justified not only according to a temporal orientation relating present time to the past (and reverse), as is often claimed, but also according to a spatial one, along relations which go from the others (neighbours, kin, etc.) to oneself. This 'horizontal' (in the sense of interrelations, not in the sense of equality) dimension of tradition-building reveals the importance of reputational mechanisms in Tajikistan, and more generally in Central Asia.

The current government, like the Soviet state before it, sees these performances of authority – be they labelled 'traditional' or 'religious' – as in competition with the authority of the state. Adept at 'secular extremism' (Lemon 2016) that targets Islamic practices, the state also performs a certain 'traditionalist authoritarianism', epitomized in recent years by the inflation of legislation and decrees that distinguish between 'good' and 'bad' tradition. The intrusive character of state decisions in the private sphere illustrates its increased endeavours to monopolize authority and to discredit any other competing figure, potentially undermining the social authority created in the realm of women's prerogatives. Yet, at least for now, the practices seem to remain stronger than any law.

Notes

1. The civil war in Tajikistan killed more than 60,000 people (1% of the population at the time) and displaced about one million people inside the country and across its borders (Kuvatova 2001). See also Ismailbekova (2015) on coping mechanisms in Kyrgyzstan.
2. On the relations between women's bodies and national projects in Central Asia, see also Cleuziou and Direnberger (2016); Ibañez-Tirado (2016); Suyarkulova (2016).
3. The term 'reputation' has the advantage, compared to 'honour', to de-exoticize social relations in Tajikistan, to separate the Tajik context from general analyses made on the basis of material from the Middle East or the Arabic world, and to better convey the meaning of my interlocutors in daily use of both Tajik words, *nomus* and *obru*.
4. For a close examination of how textiles and cosmetics reflects one's status or position, see also Ibañez-Tirado (2016).
5. Tajikistan has been until very recently the most remittance-dependent country in the world, the share of these money transfers equating 50% of its GDP (see e.g. Betti and Lundgren 2012; Buckley and Hofmann 2012; Rubinov 2016)
6. In-kind or monetary payments given in theory by the groom's family to that of the bride.
7. In-kind or monetary payments given in theory by the bride's parents to their daughter, and brought to the groom's house.
8. In-kind or monetary payments given in theory by the husband to his wife.
9. Though not everywhere. To my knowledge, people do not (yet) organize such ceremonies in the area of Gharm and Qarotegin.
10. For example, in India, see Bénéï (1995); Anderson (2007). In Vietnam, see Teerawichitchainan (2012). In China, see Siu (1993).
11. It is beyond the scope of this article to elaborate on why this reversal happened; it will be the focus of other publication. It is notable, however, that in the second half of the Soviet period, people became richer and had access to more cash but lacked ways to spend it. At the same time, bride price was targeted by the authorities as an archaic practice. The development of the dowry might have been an answer to the urge for social distinction through consumption in the context of lack of manufactured goods and ideological constraints.

12. It is possible that the Soviet ban on bride-price and the consequent stigma that it could have put on families accused of 'selling their daughters away' may have contributed to the weakening of the practice. See for example the 1967 Soviet comedy 'Kavkaskaya Plennitsa, ili Novye Priklyuchenya Shurika' (translated as 'Kidnapping, Caucasian style'), Leonid Gaïdaï's movie which mocks bride abduction and bride-price payments.
13. An important feature of dowry transfers is that they effectively consist in the repetition of unilateral gift-giving at many occasions: the bride's family makes gifts just before the wedding day, at the 'calling for the bride' after the wedding (*talbon*), at the celebration of a child's birth (*gohvora bandon*), and so on.
14. This partially explains the renewal of polygyny in the country, because being married as a second wife always seems better than not being married at all (Cleuziou 2016, 9).
15. According to Beyer, *uiat* is best translated as 'shame' only when children, who can be reprimanded directly, are concerned.
16. Although in Tajikistan spreading gossip is often women's prerogative, these examples are of women because my fieldwork took place mostly with them. But men may contribute to spreading gossip and rumours, too.
17. Full name, 'Legislative acts on the regulation of tradition, celebrations and ceremonies' (Sanadhoi me'erii huquqi oid ba tanzimi an'ana va dzhashnu marosimho). See Jumhurii Tojikiston (Republic of Tajikistan) (2007).
18. In Tajik: 'Qonuni mazkur bo taqozoi rushdi jomea an'ana va jashnu marosimho tanzim namuda, ba khifzi arzishhoi asili farhangi millii va ehtirom ba sunnathoi mardumi baroi baland bardoshtani sathi ijtimoi iqtiisodii haeti' (Jumhurii Tojikiston (Republic of Tajikistan) 2007, 6).
19. Details on the official Presidential webpage: http://www.prezident.tj/node/15923.
20. It is notable that Muslim reformists are very critical position of ceremonial spending, and have been for a long time (Dudoignon and Noack 2014). For example, conflicts exist over how weddings should proceed, and there is a tendency in certain families known for their pious background to forbid the performance of music and dance and, *a fortiori*, of lavish ceremonies. Some women have refused to participate in feasts where music is played. In the context of the crucial importance of gift-exchange in women's sociability, one can imagine the inner conflicts these decisions engender. Yet, to my knowledge, this form of celebration is not common.
21. See also the contribution of Beyer and Kojobekova (2019), in this issue.

Acknowledgments

I warmly thank Judith Beyer and Peter Finke, as well as Madeleine Reeves and the anonymous reviewers for their thoughtful comments on previous versions of this article.

Disclosure statement

No potential conflict of interest was reported by the author.

References

Abashin, S. 1999. "Kalym i Mahr v Sredney Azii. O "granytsakh" v sotsial'nykh otnoshenyakh" [Qalym and Mahr in Central Asia. On social relations boundaries], in *Chelovek i pravo*, edited by V. Tishkov and N. Novikova. Moscow: Strategiia.

Abashin, S. N. 2009. "Vopreki "zdravomu smyslu"? (K voprosy o 'racional'nosti / irracional'nosti ritualnyx rasxodov v Sredney Azii) (Against common sense? On the question of rationality or irrationality of ritual expenditure in Central Asia)." *Vestnik Evrazii* 6-7 (1-2).

Abashin, S. N. 2015. *Sovetskiĭ kishlak: Mezhdu kolonializmom i modernizat͡sieĭ.* Biblioteka zhurnala Neprikosnovennyĭ zapas (Antropologii͡a, filosofii͡a, politologii͡a, istorii͡a). Moscow: Novoe literaturnoe obozrenie.
Abrahams, R. D. 1970. "A Performance-Centred Approach to Gossip." *Man* 5 (2): 290–301. doi:10.2307/2799654.
Adams, L. L. 2010. *The Spectacular State: Culture and National Identity in Uzbekistan. Politics, History, and Culture.* Durham: Duke University Press.
Anderson, S. 2007. "The Economics of Dowry and Brideprice." *The Journal of Economic Perspectives* 21 (4): 151–174. doi: 10.2307/30033756.
Bénéï, V. 1995. "Pour une réévaluation anthropologique du 'prix de la fiancée'. Le cas du dyāj maharashtrien (Inde)", *Bulletin de l'École française d'Extrême-Orient* 82(1): 263–286. doi: 10.3406/befeo.1995.2305
Beyer, J. 2016. *The Force of Custom: Llaw and the Ordering of Everyday Life in Kyrgyzstan.* Central Eurasia in context. Pittsburgh: University of Pittsburgh Press.
Beyer, J., and A. Kojobekova. 2019. "Women of protest, men of applause: political activism, gender and tradition in Kyrgyzstan." *Central Asian Survey* 38 (3): 329–345. doi:10.1080/02634937.2019.1631258.
Betti, G., and L. Lundgren. 2012. "The Impact of Remittances and Equivalence Scales on Poverty in Tajikistan." *Central Asian Survey* 31 (4): 395–408. doi:10.1080/02634937.2012.738849.
Buckley, C., and E. T. Hofmann. 2012. "Are Remittances an Effective Mechanism for Development? Evidence from Tajikistan, 1999-2007." *Journal of Development Studies* 48 (8): 1121–1138. doi:10.1080/00220388.2012.688816.
Cleuziou, J. 2016. "'A Second Wife Is Not Really a Wife': Polygyny, Gender Relations and Economic Realities in Tajikistan." *Central Asian Survey* 35 (1): 76–90. doi:10.1080/02634937.2015.1088228.
Cleuziou, J. 2017. "Towards Matrifocal Families? Relations in Transnational and Single Parent Families in Tajikistan." In *The Family in Central Asia Past and Present: New Perspectives*, edited by S. Roche, 309–336. Berlin: K. S. Verlag.
Cleuziou, J., and L. Direnberger. 2016. "Gender and Nation in Post-Soviet Central Asia: From National Narratives to Women's Practices." *Nationalities Papers* 44 (2): 195–206. doi:10.1080/00905992.2015.1082997.
Commercio, M. E. 2015. "The Politics and Economics of "Retraditionalization" in Kyrgyzstan and Tajikistan." *Post-Soviet Affairs* 31 (6): 529–556. doi:10.1080/1060586X.2014.986870.
Danzer, A. M., B. Dietz, K. Gatskova, and A. Schmillen. 2013. "Showing off to the New Neighbors? Income, Socioeconomic Status and Consumption Patterns of Internal Migrants." 330. Working Papers. Leibniz Institut für Ost- und Südosteuropaforschung (Institute for East and Southeast European Studies). https://ideas.repec.org/p/ost/wpaper/330.html.
Direnberger, L. 2014. "Le Genre de la nation en Iran et au Tadjikistan. (Re)constructions et contestations des hétéronationalismes." (Unpublished doctoral dissertation). University Paris Diderot, Paris.
Dudoignon, S. A., and Christian Noack, eds. 2014. *Allah's Kolkhozes: Migration, de-Stalinisation, Privatisation, and the new Muslim Congregations in the Soviet Realm (1950s-2000s).* 1st ed. Islamkundliche Untersuchungen, Band 314. Berlin: KS, Klaus Schwarz Verlag.
Fathi, H. 2004. *Femmes d'autorité dans l'Asie centrale contemporaine. Quête des ancêtres et recompositions identitaires dans l'islam postsovietique.* Paris: Maisonneuve & Larose.
Harris, C. 2004. *Control and Subversion. Gender Relations in Tajikistan.* Londres: Pluto Press.
Hughes, K. 2017. "From the Achaemenids to Somoni: National Identity and Iconicity in the Landscape of Dushanbe's Capitol Complex." *Central Asian Survey* 0 (0): 1–23. doi:10.1080/02634937.2017.1319796.
Ibañez-Tirado, D. 2016. "Gold Teeth, Indian Dresses, Chinese Lycra and 'Russian' Hair: Embodied Diplomacy and the Assemblages of Dress in Tajikistan." *The Cambridge Journal of Anthropology* 34 (2): 23–41. doi:10.3167/ca.2016.340203.
Ismailbekova, A. 2015. "Single Mothers in Osh: Well-Being and Coping Strategies of Women in the Aftermath of the 2010 Conflict in Kyrgyzstan." *Focaal* 2015 (71). doi:10.3167/fcl.2015.710110.
Jumhurii Tojikiston (Republic of Tajikistan). 2007. *Sanadhoi me'yerii huquqi oid ba tanzimi an'ana va jashnu marosimho dar Jumhurii Tojikiston (Legislative acts on the regulation of tradition, celebrations and ceremonies).* Dushanbe: Republic of Tajikistan.

Kamp, M. 2006. *The New Woman in Uzbekistan: Islam, Modernity, and Unveiling Under Communism.* Washington: University of Washington Press.

Kandiyoti, D. 1988. "Bargaining With Patriarchy." *Gender and Society* 2 (3): 274–290. doi:10.1177/089124388002003004.

Kandiyoti, D. 2007. "The Politics of Gender and the Soviet Paradox: Neither Colonized, nor Modern?" *Central Asian Survey* 26 (4): 601–623. doi:10.1080/02634930802018521.

Kandiyoti, D., and N. Azimova. 2004. "The Communal and the Sacred: Women's Worlds of Ritual in Uzbekistan." *Journal of the Royal Anthropological Institute* 10 (2): 327–349. doi:10.1111/j.1467-9655.2004.00192.x.

Kisliakov, N. A. 1959. *Sem'ya i brak u Tajikov. Po materialam kontsa 19 - nachala 20 veka (Family and marriage among the Tajiks).* Vol. XLIV. Institute of Ethnography N. N. Miklukho-Maklaya. Moscow: Editions of the Academy of Sciences of USSR.

Koroteyeva, V., and E. Makarova. 1998. "Money and Social Connections in the Soviet and Post-Soviet Uzbek City." *Central Asian Survey* 17 (4): 579–596. doi:10.1080/02634939808401057.

Kuvatova, A. 2001. "Gender issues in Tajikistan: Consequences and impact of the civil war." In *Hommes armes, femmes aguerries. Rapports de genre en situations de conflict arme*, Texts gathered by Fenneke Reysoo, 127–135. Geneva: IUED.

Lemon, E. J. 2013. "Narrating Tajik History in the National Museum." *Exeter Central Asian Studies Network* (blog). 2013. http://blogs.exeter.ac.uk/excas/2013/07/24/narrating-tajik-history-in-the-national-museum/.

Lemon, E. J. 2016. "Building Resilient Secular Citizens: Tajikistan's Response to the Islamic State." *Caucasus Survey* 4 (3): 261–281. https://doi.org/10.1080/23761199.2016.1219028. doi:10.1080/23761199.2016.1219028.

McBrien, J. 2009. "Mukadas's Struggle: Veils and Modernity in Kyrgyzstan." *Journal of the Royal Anthropological Institute* 15 (may): S127–S144. doi:10.1111/j.1467-9655.2009.01546.x.

Mould, T. 2005. "The Paradox of Traditionalization: Negotiating the Past in Choctaw Prophetic Discourse." *Journal of Folklore Research: An International Journal of Folklore and Ethnomusicology* 42 (3): 255–294.

Najibullah, F., and M. Salimov. 2015. "Facebook Photos Help Convict Tajik "Birthday Boy"." *RadioFreeEurope/RadioLiberty*, 25 August 2015, sect. Tajikistan. http://www.rferl.org/content/tajikistan-facebook-used-to-convict-birthday-boy/27208345.html.

Nalivkin, V., and M. Nalivkina. 1886. *Očerk byta ženščiny osědlago tuzemnago naseleniâ Fergany (Report on the life of women in the native sedentary population of the Ferghana).* Kazan: Edition of Imperial University.

Nourzhanov, K. 2001. "The Politics of History in Tajikistan: Reinventing the Samanids." *Harvard Asia Quarterly* 5 (1): 21–30.

Origgi, G. 2015. *La réputation: qui dit quoi de qui.* 1st ed. Paris: PUF.

Petric, B.-M., 2004. *Pouvoir, don et réseaux en Ouzbékistan postsoviétique.* Paris: PUF.

Poliakov, S. P. 1992. *Everyday Islam: Religion and Tradition in Rural Central Asia.* Armonk, NY: Routledge.

Reeves, M. 2012. "Black Work, Green Money: Remittances, Ritual, and Domestic Economies in Southern Kyrgyzstan." *Slavic Review* 71: 108–138. doi:10.5612/slavicreview.71.1.0108.

Roche, S. 2014. *Domesticating Youth: Youth Bulges and its Socio-Political Implications in Tajikistan.* Integration and conflict studies, vol. 8. New York: Berghahn.

Roche, S. 2015. "Twenty-Five Somonis for a Good Future: How Young Women in Tajikistan Shape Their Futures and Secure Their Present." *Central Asian Affairs* 2: 71–94. doi:10.1163/22142290-00201005.

Roche, S. 2016. "A Sound Family for a Healthy Nation: Motherhood in Tajik National Politics and Society." *Nationalities Papers* 44 (2): 207–224. doi:10.1080/00905992.2015.1087486.

Rubinov I., 2016. *The Impact of Migration and Remittances on Natural Resources in Tajikistan.* Center for International Forestry Research, Occasional Paper 164. http://www.cifor.org/…/OP-164.pdf

Schechner, R. 2013. *Performance Studies: An Introduction.* London: Routledge.

Siu, H. 1993. "Reconstituting Dowry and Brideprice in South China." In *Chinese Families in the Post-Mao Era*, edited by D. Davis and D. Harrell, 165–188. Berkeley: University of California Press.

Stephan, M. 2010. "Education, Youth and Islam: The Growing Popularity of Private Religious Lessons in Dushanbe, Tajikistan." *Central Asian Survey* 29 (4): 469–483. doi:10.1080/02634937.2010.538283.
Stephan-Emmrich, M., and A. Mirzoev. 2016. "The Manufacturing of Islamic Lifestyles in Tajikistan Through the Prism of Dushanbe's Bazaars." *Central Asian Survey* 35 (2): 157–177. doi:10.1080/02634937.2016.1152008.
Suyarkulova, M. 2016. "Fashioning the Nation: Gender and Politics of Dress in Contemporary Kyrgyzstan." *Nationalities Papers* 44 (2): 247–265. doi:10.1080/00905992.2016.1145200.
Sukhareva, O. 1940. "Svadebnye obrâdy Tağikov g. Samarkanda i nekotoryx drugyx rajonov Srednej Azii." *Sovietskaâ Etnografiâ* III: 172–176.
Teerawichitchainan, B., 2012. "Tradition and Change in Marriage Payments in Vietnam, 1963–2000." *Asian Population Studies* 8(2): 151-172. doi: 10.1080/17441730.2012.675677.
Tett, G. 1996. "Ambiguous Alliances Marriage and Identity in a Muslim Village in Soviet Tajikistan." (Unpublished Ph.D. dissertation). University of Cambridge, Cambridge.
Thibault, H. 2013. "The Secular and the Religious in Tajikistan: Contested Political Spaces." *Studies in Religion/Sciences Religieuses* 42 (2): 173–189. doi:10.1177/0008429813479297.
Trevisani, T. 2016. "Modern Weddings in Uzbekistan: Ritual Change from 'above' and from 'Below'." *Central Asian Survey* 35 (1): 61–75. doi:10.1080/02634937.2015.1114781.
Werner, C. 2009. "Bride Abduction in Post-Soviet Central Asia: Marking a Shift Towards Patriarchy Through Local Discourses of Shame and Tradition." *Journal of the Royal Anthropological Institute* 15 (2): 314–331. doi:10.1111/j.1467-9655.2009.01555.x.
Yuval-Davis, N. 1993. "Gender and Nation." *Ethnic and Racial Studies* 16 (4): 621–632. doi:10.1080/01419870.1993.9993800.
Zelizer, V. A. 2000. "The Purchase of Intimacy." *Law & Social Inquiry* 25 (3): 817–848. doi:10.1111/j.1747-4469.2000.tb00162.x.

The body global and the body traditional: a digital ethnography of Instagram and nationalism in Kazakhstan and Russia

Diana T. Kudaibergenova

ABSTRACT

What is the power of social media in defining and policing sexual identities and bodily expressions, and what are their connections to understanding nation, power and self in authoritarian contexts? Through the study of popular Instagram accounts in Kazakhstan and Russia, I argue that these sites serve as spaces of visualization and re-creation of new forms of 'acceptable' behaviour and lifestyles, that on the one hand may lead to new globalized visions of sexual identity and the body while on the other promoting localized conflict and resentment online, triggered by online users' fear of losing their 'national culture' in these global trends. While many resort to policing gender norms and heteronormative body images online, influencers and Instagrammers from Russia and Kazakhstan take an active part in resisting these frameworks and categories.

Introduction

In the last 10 years, social media have come to play an important role in shaping norms and codes of practice all over the world. Social media are used for interpersonal communication and information seeking. Platforms such as Facebook, Twitter, Snapchat, and Instagram provide users with information and allow them to track new trends and connect with new people, but also to acquiesce to surveillance (Sheldon and Bryant 2016), monitoring and the stigmatization of behaviour. Given their impact on society, social media have been studied already with regard to their links to the emergence and transformation of norms and values (Olszanowski 2014; Carr and Hayes 2015; Pearce and Vitak 2015; Tiidenberg 2015; Duguay 2016). Social media like Instagram shape consumption and beauty standards and serve as an influential platform for the discussion of all sorts of identities, from gender to national and traditional identities and worldviews. The scholarly literature on social media already includes such important topics as bodily representations (Lupton 2017; Santarossa and Woodruff 2017), race (Cirucci 2017), class, and gender and sexuality (Duffy and Hund 2015; Burgess et al. 2016; Duguay 2016). Gender, sexuality, the influence of dating apps, virtual mobbing, and the creation of virtual worlds of relationships, scandals and battles across the world by people who may never see each other face to face, have already influenced the ways we study new social interactions online. The study of social media also helps us understand trends in national identities through global digitalized networks and communications.

Central Asia is part of these global discussions, where the influence of social media on the everyday lives of its citizens and communities is increasingly felt. When Kyrgyz feminist and singer Zere Asylbek's video 'Kyz' (Girl) went viral in September 2018, it instantly spread across thousands of Central Asian social media accounts, with comments and instant 'sharing' in different languages. Only after that did the video and the discourse of female liberation and equal rights for all women for which it advocated enter the realm of more traditional media through the singer's subsequent interviews and podcasts.[1] Zere's online popularity shed light on how certain messages and discourses could reach wider audiences. But it is also online and in the realm of social media that feminist liberation meets harsh opposition from the discourses of those who strive to control new understandings of 'tradition' and 'shame' locally. This is visible in the narrative of the so-called 'uyat-men' (*uyat* means shame) that preceded Zere's success and became popular due to the spread of social media use globally and in the region.

In March 2016, Talgat Sholtayev, who lives in Kazakhstan's capital, Astana, decided to cover one of the statues on the city's central boulevard with a throw. The statue, which was installed in the centre of Astana in 2005, represented two young people, a woman and a man, in love. The work of Kazakh sculptor Tolepbai Erbolat did not attract much interest until one blogger complained of the female figure's 'nudity', with its clear features of breasts, nipples and buttocks. Sholtayev, who gave himself the name 'Uyat-man', found the sculpture 'offensive' to Kazakh traditions and covered the female statue with a throw; he then posted a picture of himself next to it on Facebook (Figure 1).[2]

Through this photo, the term 'uyat-man' became for some a symbol of cosmopolitan resistance and a means to critique tradition and traditional values, and for others the ground to justify retraditionalizing practices. If traditionalization is the process of following

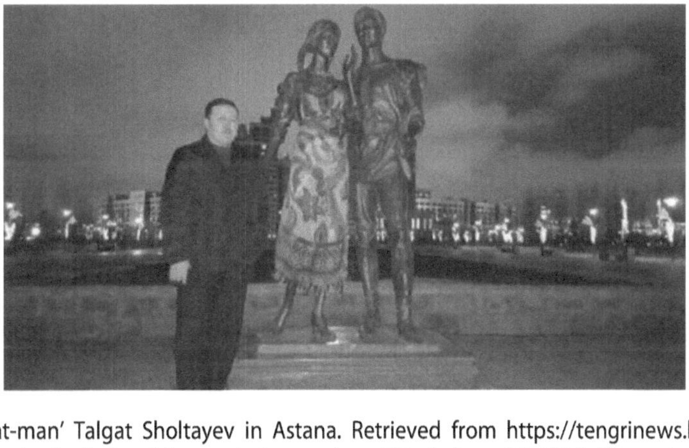

Figure 1. 'Uyat-man' Talgat Sholtayev in Astana. Retrieved from https://tengrinews.kz/kazakhstan_news/jitel-astanyi-nakryil-skandalnuyu-skulpturu-devushki-platkom-290828/. The author and the publishers have made their best endeavours to trace the copyright holder of this image. The publisher welcomes communications from the copyright holder, so that the appropriate acknowledgements can be made.

certain traditional and often patriarchal ways of living established and legitimated by the community who lives by them, then retraditionalization is understood here as a powerful and power-seeking discourse about one's culture, nation and tradition in the wake of globalization and growing nationalism. Through retraditionalization, actors seek to establish power over defining what 'national tradition' means, by rethinking tradition in a more contemporary sense, for example by arguing that bride kidnapping is a romanticized discourse of love and freedom (Kudaibergenova 2017). In this context, shaming is often used as a legitimation for maintaining a so-called or imagined 'traditional' order that more generally represents heterosexual normative behaviour more than anything else. *Uyat* (shame) is also deep-seated in this matrix of retraditionalizing practices and power-seeking activities through online shaming.

The discourse of *uyat* that evolved as a consequence of Sholtayev's actions became so popular that it has already resulted in one popular theatrical play, numerous blog posts, an Internet meme, a graphic novel and a video game, with Uyat-man as the protagonist.[3] In the game, Uyat-man comes and covers topless Kazakh ladies who share their semi-naked photos online (Figure 2). In the imagination of numerous online users and popular local meme creators, Uyat-man also follows young women to the beaches where they pose in bikinis, and even invades art museums to cover other naked female statues – not just in Kazakhstan but world-wide.

What is at the heart of these discussions is the body and its socially acceptable or unacceptable behaviour, as well as the visualization and censorship of images depicting naked, sexualized, objectified, national and nationalized, traditional and retraditionalized bodies. The body has long been described as a site of power struggles in social theory (Foucault 1990; Featherstone, Hepworth, and Turner 1991; Turner 2008), and more vocally in gender studies (Young 1990; Yuval-Davis 1997; Fournier 2002). The body is the focal point of these controlling mechanisms. It is simultaneously the nationalized and the gendered body; it also becomes the space where heterosexual norms are imposed and controlled through discourses of 'appropriate behaviour' collectively imagined in the name of the nation. But not all groups agree to these collectively established ideas of 'appropriate behaviour', even if they live within the limits and discourses of the same nation. As I will demonstrate, bodies exposed on Instagram are open to varying discourses and controlling practices by

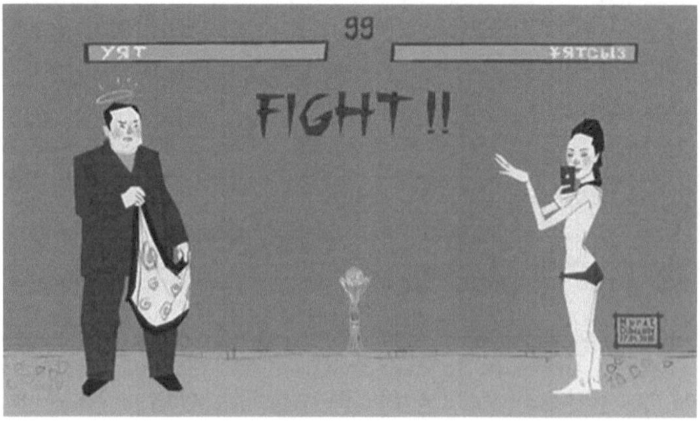

Figure 2. Uyat/Uyatssyz video game, April 2016. Image © Murat Dilmanov

external agents. These agents strongly believe that shaming someone else's body is done in the name and for the national cultural values that they continuously redefine. Instagram has become a lively visual-based online community for debating these views and discourses where users can easily connect through their mobile phones and from anywhere in the world.

Instagram is the fastest-growing social media site in the world (Sheldon and Bryant 2016) and the most popular social medium among people under 29 worldwide (Pew Research 2016).[4] Instagram is a phone or computer application where users have to register and create their own profile before they start connecting with other people through a network of hashtags and *publics* (digital communities). Unlike other social media such as Facebook or Twitter, Instagram is picture-based and video-based only. It is highly popular in Russia, where almost 30% of Russian internet users were registered on Instagram in 2016,[5] and it is also the fastest-growing mobile app in Kazakhstan, where an estimated of 3.3–4.3 million Kazakhstanis (out of 17 million) use social media such as Instagram daily.[6]

In this article I draw on the existing literature on the body, viewing it as a battlefield for gendered norms, disciplining practices and traditionalist inscriptions through the mechanisms of cyber-bullying, 'slut-shaming' and framing non-traditional (non-heterosexual) sexual behaviour as unacceptable on Instagram. Through digital ethnography of Instagram-based discourses and discussions, I explore how this global social media site simultaneously promotes globalized perspectives on gender norms and sexuality and at the same time reinforces practices of traditionalization.

Nationalizing regimes and online discourses

My discussion in this article is framed in the context of fluid cultural perceptions in the increasingly authoritarian conditions of the two biggest post-Soviet states, Russia and Kazakhstan. Both countries embrace neoliberal norms of mass consumption and the objectification of the body, yet in both states there is a simultaneous trend towards traditionalist and nationalist attacks on individual freedoms (Makarychev and Medvedev 2015; Kudaibergenova 2017, 2018). In Russia and Kazakhstan, heterosexual norms are invoked with a contextual and individual understanding of 'national culture' that needs to be defended from globalized norms shared online (Tiidenberg 2015; Mamedov 2016; Rodulgina 2016; Stella and Nartova 2016). Authoritarianism, defined by the lack of alternative views and pluralism and guided by the decisions of the inner circle of ruling political elites, feeds back into limiting nationalist discourse and traditionalist perspectives on gender and the body.

Both Russia and Kazakhstan are nationalizing regimes where power elites seek to establish order and control over powerful and meaningful discourses that guide social order on what the core narrative of the nation means. Nationalizing regimes seek to establish control over debates concerning the body which come to serve as a stand-in for the national unity of their respective states (Kudaibergenova 2016). As Stella and Nartova (2016, 19) argue, in Russia,

> the ruling political elites have sought to appropriate the narrative of national unity and national interest in order to create order, build consensus and strengthen their dwindling legitimacy in a deeply divided society, fraught with gaping social inequalities and interethnic tensions.

In Kazakhstan, a similar process followed, where (former) president Nursultan A. Nazarbayev's nationalizing regime aimed to create a comprehensive umbrella of discourses concerning the Kazakh nation and interethnic harmony under what I call a compartmentalized ideology, where the president himself legitimizes his power as the only guarantor of inter-ethnic peace, economic development and stability in the country (Kudaibergenova 2016, 2019). Traditionalist discourses of controlling heterosexual norms fall under these desires to keep order enshrined in the discursive understanding of power, nation and gender.

This desire to control and create a heterosexual normative order clashes with the discourses shared on global social media such as Instagram. This is why many regimes aim to control social media and online spaces, for example, in China and during the Arab Spring in Egypt (Bamman, O'Connor, and Smith 2012; Castells 2015). Certain states seek to establish tighter control of social media because 'as the communications landscape gets denser, more complex, and more participatory, the networked population is gaining greater access to information, more opportunities to engage in public speech, and an enhanced ability to undertake collective action' (Shirky 2011, 29; see also Lewis 2016 on blogging in Kazakhstan).

Retraditionalization discourses have become tools for the collective targeting and shaming of 'deviant' discourses online. In this article I focus on three instances of sexualization and 'slut-shaming': homosexuality as a direct deviation from heteronormativity; transsexuality; and bodily liberation. In the following discussion I analyze the online presence of three popular Instagram bloggers: Madina Musina (known as Mada Mada) and Diana Idris from Kazakhstan; and Aadya (name changed) from Russia.

My choice of cases follows the hypothesis that traditionalist discourses and retraditionalizing practices would attack what these critics perceive as 'globalized' sets of behaviours: female promiscuity or sexual liberation and queerness. I chose all three bloggers after having interacted with them frequently on Instagram since the autumn of 2013, witnessing the rise of their popularity online.[7] Mada Mada made a name for herself as a vocal supporter of the 'body positive' movement. Diana Idris rose to popularity after her mockery of the traditionalist and patronizing behaviours of mothers-in-law in Kazakhstan. Aadya, who claims to be the first openly transgender person in Russia, expanded her online audiences after a 'slut-shaming' group that focuses on exposing sex workers uploaded her photo along with her Instagram credentials in the autumn of 2013. These bloggers openly attack traditionalist discourses, bringing the debate over globalized and traditionalist views in Kazakhstan and Russia to the height of popular online discussion on Instagram. All three accounts also expose some of the most discussed photos, videos, and more recently Instagram stories (videos and highlights that last only for one day). While there are many more popular bloggers on Instagram, their content focuses more on consumption and 'beauty blogging', that is advertising beauty products and clothing brands. The focus of my study is on the clash of globalized and retraditionalized perceptions of the body, and in this debate Madina Musina, Diana Idris and Aadya provide the most vocal and heated discussions and stories.

A digital ethnography of Instagram: likes, hashtags, comments and publics

There are many ways to study social media, but digital ethnography proves to be the most effective tool, since this type of ethnography allows one to focus on alternative views and platforms that are located online. Digital ethnography tells stories and analyzes social interactions not through the realm of face-to-face communication but through virtual communication in the form of comment boxes, blogging and sharing of content, both pictorial and verbal. Digital ethnography 'combines a wide lens and a microscopic attention to detail', and thus 'it is perfect for capturing environments and their contexts but also the microdynamics that produce them' (Madianou 2016, 2). Digital ethnography is defined in the growing field of social media studies as

> a method for representing real-life cultures through combining the characteristic features of digital media with the elements of story. These projects use the expressive and procedural potential of computer-based storytelling to enable audiences to go beyond absorbing facts about another culture to entering into the experience of that culture. (Underberg and Zorn 2013, 10)

Digital research on cultures allows flexibility in space and encounter with such cultures but also focuses on different and at times unexpected and unconventional studies of culture. It is not located in a physical space, but rather the notion of culture travels across the different cases once these are located online. For example, a Russian blogger might reach audiences anywhere in the world without having to physically travel (or stay in Moscow). The question of language does matter on Instagram, where local bloggers often write in their local languages, in my case Russian and Kazakh. But since the content on Instagram is mainly picture- and video-based, linguistic capabilities often do not create major problems, as many users often leave comments in their own languages or rely on automatic translation. Many popular bloggers write either in English or in both Russian and English. The popular Russian Instagram blogger Miroslava Duma (1.6 million followers) mainly writes in English, while Lena Perminova (1.8 million followers) writes in both English and Russian, and former Russian presidential candidate Xenia Sobchak (5.9 million followers) writes mainly in Russian.

On Instagram, users communicate by uploading their videos and pictures and then connecting through the use of hashtags (#) to attract more attention to any particular topic. Hashtag mapping is a methodology that was used for the study of Twitter (Bruns and Burgess 2011; Instagram, Terms of Use n.d.); it employs 'the filtering of the collected data based on time and keywords' (Highfield and Leaver 2015, 2). In my digital ethnography, which started in autumn 2013 and lasted until January 2019, I visited Instagram regularly, four or five times a day, to check for new comments and stories. However, this type of qualitative search and tracking requires selecting the targeted bloggers or hashtags in advance. This was the initial step taken in the first six months of the research (April to October 2013), preceding the first presentation of the initial data in October 2013. After the first phase I identified three targeted bloggers and followed them thoroughly and daily from October 2013 until November 2018.

To identify the targeted bloggers, I searched through the hashtags associated with relevant keywords, such as #queer, #sex, #Kazakhstan, #uyat [shame], #beautyblogger and #Russia (in both Russian and English languages). I started scouting for popular local publics, that is digital communities based on common interests. A public is an account set up by one or many individuals who act as editors. The followers of any specific public use it to share information, and to comment on things that are interesting to them. Many companies or lobby groups establish publics on Instagram to attract attention to their activities. But popular publics mostly provide entertaining content – trendy videos, funny jokes, memes, fashion trends – and often include controversial and pressing issues, such as discussions of promiscuity, traditional marriage, love, and sex life in general.

In 2013 I found that Koten-Insta (which no longer exists) and ZTB (Za_Tebya_Bake or For_You_Bake) were some of the most popular publics, Koten-Insta having more than 50,000 followers and ZTB currently having almost 100,000. Both names have a local flavour. Koten-Insta is a combination of the Kazakh word for 'butt' with a popular nickname for Instagram, Insta. 'For You, Bake' is also a localized Kazakh colloquial saying, where Bake is a nickname for the male name Baken.

In Russia, Labuten_vsemu_golova ('Louboutin is the head of everything', the public that specialized in exposing sex workers on social media) was one of the most popular publics, with 3000 comments in the first 15 minutes of sharing a new picture in 2013–2014. I chose to follow two publics, Koten-Insta in Kazakhstan and Labuten_vsemu_golova in Russia, for 12 months, from autumn 2013 to autumn 2014. The main aim of these two publics was to target and shame people for their 'deviant' or non-heteronormative behaviour, which in turn also became the focus of my study.[8]

It was impossible to trace who the editor(s) of these publics were or how they generated their content. At one-point Koten-Insta announced their contact information on WhatsApp (another social media platform) for anyone interested in sharing content. The editor(s) then selected what they perceived to be the best content and posted it to their Instagram account. Labuten_vsemu_golova similarly followed their viewers' suggestions through hashtags when users were tagging specific Instagram accounts (mainly women) whom they considered sex workers hiding behind a 'beauty blogger' title. In what followed, the editor(s) of Labuten_vsemu_golova claimed they contacted these beauty bloggers and published their conversations, in which the beauty blogger allegedly offered their sex services in exchange for money. Labuten_vsemu_golova specialized in 'filtering' and exposing (Russ. *vyvesti na chistuyu vodu*; lit. to bring into clear water) these bloggers. These posts received the most likes.[9] But there was no further verification that this information about the beauty bloggers being sex workers was true.

When I started following this public, in autumn 2013, there was an ongoing scandal regarding the sharing of a video of a popular female blogger whom they had exposed, naked and in expensive outfits, accompanied by a derogatory song.[10] Many users tagged the female blogger who was exposed in this video, and she tried to block Labuten_vsemu_golova from sharing it. But instead she had to delete her own Instagram account after Labuten_vsemu_golova followers and editor(s) continued to cyber-bully her by exposing her real name, posting alleged prices for her sex work services, and even making fun of her husband and child.[11] All of that spurred a lot of scandal online at the time, but it did not stop Labuten_vsemu_golova and similar publics from continuously 'exposing' women whose pictures and videos they found on Instagram. Eventually, Labuten_vsemu_golova shared a picture of Aadya, shaming her for being Muslim, for being from the Caucasus and for being openly transgender. This is how I started following her, as many followers of Labuten_vsemu_golova tagged her Instagram account in their comments on the picture. Around the same time, Koten-Insta shared a video by Diana Idris where she rapped about second wives (Kaz.: *toqals*). By that time, I had already followed the Kazakhstan Internet sensation, Madina Musina, who called for a boycott of female virginity tests, which had been in unofficial use to prove that young women had not engaged in premarital sex. The virginity test involves a visit to a gynaecologist.

In this digital ethnography of Instagram, I also used my own network of followed pages and bloggers to connect with people. At first, this included popular female and male lifestyle bloggers, feminists and LGBTQ activists across different post-Soviet countries, but Russia and Kazakhstan provided most of content. I observed discussions and followed a number of popular groups and bloggers, which formed part of the digital ethnography. Due to the frequency with which comments were removed, I had to check and collect the digital data for comments, photos and posts multiple times per day and to save screenshots on my laptop. Social media research is a new field for researchers worldwide, and it requires ethical treatment of privacy (Olszanowski 2014; Carr and Hayes 2015; Duffy and Hund 2015; Pearce and Vitak 2015; Tiidenberg 2015; Burgess et al. 2016; Duguay 2016; Cirucci 2017; Lupton 2017; Santarossa and Woodruff 2017). All the accounts I followed were and are open to the public, which means that they can become the target of surveillance, stalking or cyber-bullying. I therefore do not reveal names or photos of the people I studied, instead focusing on content and discussions that the content of these pages spurred.

The limitations of Instagram provide only a ban of the account but no legal prosecution, since the latter is dependent on local, country-based legal precedents.[12] These conditions create a situation wherein users are not directly protected by the social media platform from possible defamation or critique. The only measure that can be taken is to delete an account or the specific defaming content. In late January 2018, one of the accounts publicly shared screenshots from a zoophilic adult film featuring a young woman who resembled one of the popular Instagram bloggers. People who shared screenshots followed Instagram's conventional rules of covering female nipples and private parts but left the face and the presumed action visible. They also posted the Instagram name of the female blogger whom they assumed performed in this video and widely shared it online. The female blogger was forced to close her popular Instagram account, and several hours later the screenshots of the video with her name also disappeared from the 'shaming' Instagram account. However, even after such grave, unethical actions over something they cannot provide proof of, the Labuten_vsemu_golova Instagram public, which shared and reproduced this story, was not deleted or suspended, but only gained even more followers. Eventually, Labuten_vsemu_golova's popularity diminished, and when I checked it again two years later, it had lost most of its followers because its content was too often banned.

While my example of the two publics is rather extreme, similar discussions develop on personal Instagram accounts. Overall, the platform remains a space for constant power struggles over the definition of what is appropriate and what is not in a given 'culture' or country. This example reveals that while some use Instagram to invoke 'tradition' as a means to promote patriarchal and heteronormative discourses, for others it constitutes an empowering space to oppose these very same discourses.

Sex, sexualization and fat: all the things that women are not supposed to talk about

In Kazakhstan, Madina Musina, known as Mada Mada (or Devochka Kolbasa, now Lady Kolbasa on Instagram), became the most popular feminist online blogger through her struggle to lose weight. She tackled the standards of radicalized beauty, domestic violence, family relations and gender stereotypes that are often exposed on social media

(Lupton 2017; Santarossa and Woodruff 2017). Her book *Zhir*, an abbreviation of 'woman looking for rationality' (*zhenshina, ishushyaya ratsional'nost*) that also reads as 'fat' in Russian, became a bestseller. In it she shares her memories and thoughts of being a woman in a patriarchal society.[13] Twenty-four-year old Madina Musina, who grew up in Almaty and spent some of her teen years in the US, often uses her cosmopolitan views and does not hide her love of globalization. She quickly attracted attention to her account with her discussions of bodily fat and love of food as a 'real Central Asian woman'. When I started following Madina Musina in the autumn of 2013, she was posting pictures of herself in Uzbek *ikat* silk dresses and gossiping about 'handsome waiters' at local Uzbek restaurants. At the same time, she shared stories of her 'mixed' ethnic background (Tatar, Uzbek and Kazakh) and criticized Kazakh nationalism. As a result, she became famous – a so-called Instagram 'influencer' who has over 100,000 followers on Instagram alone.[14]

At first glance her account represents a battle against the gendered and racial stereotypes to which she was subjected. Her choice of photographs shows her as a happy young girl, as a teenager and as a young woman. Under each picture, she has sarcastic comments about her 'non-ideal body shape', sometimes giving the actual number of kilos she weighed at the time. With these posts, Madina Musina unleashed criticism and comments but also elicited messages about bodily politics and liberated sexuality. These photos represent a good-looking young woman with excessive make-up, strong full red lips and frank sarcasm in her eyes. Madina Musina wrote about her love life and her family relations and offered advice on how to deal with related problems in these areas. In 2019, she became involved in youth protests in Almaty, adding political reviews to her posts on her personal life.

The words and themes Madina Musina chose in the beginning of her discussions were not gentle or customary to those of her followers who supported traditionalist discourses. But her followers continued to follow her because of the popular content she was sharing, because they enjoyed reading her texts or fighting with her, and because she is an influencer. Madina Musina often cursed, sometimes inventing her own words to avoid internet censorship, used sexualized jargon and portrayed herself as a diva. She also positioned herself as a feminist, anti-nationalist and anti-*uyat* blogger. For instance, she proposed to celebrate women's first day of menstruation in a manner similar to the celebration of male circumcisions that are widely and proudly practiced in Central Asia. 'Why not celebrate young girls in the same manner?' Madina Musina wrote on her Instagram, under a photo that celebrated an affluent young female friend dancing in a nightclub in 2017. The same post was duplicated on her Facebook page and was criticized by many. She followed these criticisms with a post about oral sex and invited even more criticisms with her 'rhetorical question', 'do you think Kazakh women do not perform oral sex?'

Sex and the accompanying norms regarding what a Kazakh woman is allowed and not allowed to do have been on Madina Musina's agenda since she began using Instagram. A post on her Instagram page from 26 October 2015 reads:

> Dear girls! Please save your virginity as the biggest treasure [that you have]! Put it in a red velvet cushion inside a little glass box. Safeguard your virginity because it is the most important thing in the world otherwise your husband would never forgive you [for not being a

> virgin on the first night after the wedding] and you will dishonour [yourself and your family]! It is shameful! [Don't have sex] before marriage! P.S. But it is ok to perform [oral] sex and anal sex.

In summer 2017 she raised eyebrows among her critics when she started a campaign for people to pray for her own next sexual encounter since she had broken up with her last boyfriend and felt lonely and depressed. On 5 August 2017 she then posted a happy note on her Facebook page announcing her positive sexual endeavour, with a picture of her followers crossing their fingers for her for good luck, and the note:

> Guys, it worked! If you really want something, make 230 people cross their fingers for you. I had sex. I came alive. And I had been suffering because of one [man] like a [stupid] sheep while there are so many cool men around!!!

When one male Facebook user shared and criticized her posts being about 'each of her shags' and recommended sarcastically that Madina Musina 'share [her] biorhythms and address with others so they can join you', an implicit threat, she mocked him. Musina's online presence was and continues to be a manifestation of a new way of doing things for some very liberal women in Kazakhstan, but it did not touch on the more general problems of gender domination. Musina became a symbol of new young liberated woman for many in social media of Kazakhstan.

Putting 'traditional' roles on display – weddings, big celebrations and parties (Kaz.: *toi*) – Diana Idris also claimed her fame through Instagram, where she shared her disenchantment with the 'puff' of big Kazakh wedding celebrations. She comes from the southern city of Shymkent and often shares her posts in the Kazakh language, directly targeting 'typical' Kazakh lifestyles, goals and values that are stereotypically 'traditional' in her view. Examples include the despotic mother-in-law relationships with her *kelin* (daughter-in-law) or the aspirations of 'little Kazakh men' – Astana-based clerks dreaming about their big future in government. Idris is sarcastic about these values, but in contrast to Madina Musina's experience, Idris embodies her 'traditional' roles as a former daughter-in-law, and as an ex-wife who had to go through 'needless *toi*' – celebrations of her wedding – as well as the domestic violence that followed soon after. In one of her Instagram posts, which is related to her future book, she openly wrote that all of the roles she has come to represent are still parts of her own self.

Thus, Diana Idris, unlike Madina Musina, had already embraced her 'traditional' role in her personal life during eight years of marriage in Shymkent, where, in her own words, she was a 'professional *kelin*' (daughter-in-law, see Kudaibergenova 2018) and wore a headscarf as a symbol of her marriage.[15] In her own words, she considered the 'traditional' attire of Shymkent *kelins* – a formless dress and a headscarf – an 'adventurous quest' and had to learn to 'survive in a patriarchal society' by growing manly inside. Idris embodies resistance to practices of traditionalization in that she fashions herself as a survivor. This is why her Instagram account is so popular. She openly contests and ridicules the traditionally powerful mothers-in-law (*ene*) and powerless daughters-in-law (*kelin*), as well as the position of second wives (*toqal*), who have become more popular in Kazakhstan in the last years, showing that retraditionalization can go hand in hand with economic opportunities and a more global way of life brought about by labour migration. The popularity of second wives or *toqals* is often justified in Kazakhstan by the popularity or rather subjective reading of Islamic texts, whereas in reality, it is a sign of further patriarchization of the society that Idris criticizes.

Like Madina Musina's posts, Idris's online presence invites a lot of criticism but also support. Both sets of followers have grown rapidly, and she has been invited to TV shows as a commentator on such issues as women's rights and marriage.

It comes as no surprise that members of this new wave of feminism in Kazakhstan use the internet and social media as their main source and ground for work as a space still relatively free of state control and censorship. But unfortunately, social media does not empower everyone equally. This discourse remains within the frames of an ethnic 'Kazakh' domain, although most of the materials about gendered problems and stereotypes are published in Russian. And while many of these discourses do incorporate the rights of LGBTQ communities, and although all the feminist bloggers, including Madina Musina and Diana Idris, are advocates for the rights of those identifying as LGBTQ, these themes remain marginalized, even when the blogger is transsexual.[16]

In my final case study, I analyze an example of bodily liberation to show how traditionalized practices influence the free choice of a transgender woman who came from the religious and cultural context of the Russian Caucasus. Aadya's story and Instagram success are important here as she is one of the most vocal transgender voices not just in Russia but across post-Soviet space.

Bodily and sexual liberation

Aadya, a transsexual blogger from Russia, is very open about her transition experience despite growing transphobia and physical threats to her in her own country, which is why I chose to anonymize her name. I found her account through the public that shared two photos of her: Aadya as a man and as a woman after transition. Every year on 31 March she celebrates International Transgender Day of Visibility by posting photos of her transition from a male to a female body, even though the trans movement in Russia is fairly new (Kirey-Sitnikova 2016). Her Instagram account is also dedicated to her liberating 'bodily' experience. Every photo of her in what her followers call a 'naked dress' (Russ. *goloe platie*) is a tribute to liberty, femininity and success.

Despite her constantly changing her Instagram account, she has a stable following of 20,000–40,000. Aadya is famous in Russia, and as a very attractive woman who is not ashamed of her sexuality she talks openly about her multiple lovers and even posts photos of their torsos and tattoos on her page, only to take them down due to ongoing scandals, including issues of privacy and visibility. She also frequently had to take down her own photos in 2016, as pictures of her (usually naked) body and nipples violated Instagram's guidelines on female nudity. Instead, she started posting more photos of her gym practice and explained how she achieved such a feminine body after her plastic surgery, including sex reassignment surgery. Aadya focused on her surgery in detail for her Instagram followers in a number of posts, but when new followers asked her personal questions about her sex life, she answered them openly. She never hid her previous self and admitted that it is still a part of her. On numerous occasions, she addressed her critics by pointing out that it was not her choice to be born as a man and that she regretted not being able to bear children as a woman.

Aadya's Instagram account, like those of other bloggers discussed in this article, was not envisioned as a platform for LGBTQ rights but rather aimed at attracting attention to herself, depicting her everyday lifestyle in ways that might be interesting to other people. With her growing popularity, it is also unusual that she does not monetize her Instagram by promoting products, as other famous fashion or lifestyle bloggers do. Her influence on Instagram cannot be overestimated.

One of her recurrent narratives of self-development concerns beauty standards. Aadya shared her story and photos of a lip implant she had to replace and wrote about her breast implants. In these posts, she blamed stereotypical views about female beauty as the main reason for her early and naive views on how to transform her body. Now she advocates natural and attainable beauty standards, healthy food and regular workouts. Many of her followers (mainly young women) accept her as a role model and share comments of admiration. These same female followers attack the 'haters' and cyber-bullies who post negative and discriminatory posts.

Through her Instagram narratives, Aadya represents herself as a strong person, reflecting on her North Caucasus roots and her traditional upbringing. From time to time, she even shares posts in her native language or writes about her understanding of values and traditions or religion. The main idea behind these posts and Aadya's own position regarding religiosity and tradition is that tradition can take over one's freedom (of expression). In her rare snapshots of life before her bodily transformation she compares it to the worst torture, not being able 'to be who you truly are'. So, when someone tries to 'bring her back to her senses' by labelling her a 'traditional Caucasus' man or woman who is supposed to display manly features or behave like a chaste woman, she bans these people and writes another post about her liberation and her right as a person to do what she pleases.

Aadya's sex life and attitudes, which come as a background to her whole profile on Instagram, are seen by some of her followers as a problem. Aadya openly discusses her love life. Since she decided to 'enjoy life', in her own words, and became a liberated woman, some call her a slut (Russian: *rasputnaya zhenshina*). Aadya makes no secret of her sexual preferences and desires and finds potential suitors online and in Moscow bars. According to her posts, they have to be young, good-looking and insatiable. Her relations are brief and public on Instagram. On her Instagram account Aadya presents herself as a person who was suppressed by cultural, religious, and moral forces for a long time and who now wants to channel her full rejection of shame publicly, since the public aspect of shame is its biggest power.

In this narration of self-liberation and resistance to being shamed, the body becomes a site of empowerment. In repressive conditions of public shaming, including 'slut-shaming' and body shaming, the body itself is separated from the self and is presented and exposed as a powerless object of gaze and judgement, vulnerable to attacks from the outside. By taking back control of their bodies by means of such visual sites as Instagram, bloggers like Aadya and Madina Musina take back power over themselves, their decisions and their lifestyles. The body is also clearly linked to sexual preferences as a physical site of pleasure and desire. One's decision to go against the set norms of heteronormativity and to seek pleasure from the same-sex body is also an act of self-empowerment and resistance to the dominant power of these norms.

The *uyat* discourse as a norm-setting tool

Returning to the discourse of shame, in the last part of this article I show how practices of retraditionalization work in combination with social media and globalized networks. Following Beyer and Finke (2019), I argue that while practices of traditionalization might be frequently linked to supposedly old perceptions and beliefs in sacred traditions that represent a patriarchal traditionalist agenda (Kudaibergenova 2017, 2018), it is more fruitful to understand 'traditionalization as a bottom-up process in which elites do not necessarily dictate the course of events, let alone the outcomes' (Beyer and Finke 2019, 2). Taking the example of Uyat-man (shaming man), who became a popular culture meme and a trend in Kazakhstan, I show how this trend has influenced further discussions of retraditionalization and globalization online in Kazakhstan. The activities of Uyat-man built on practices that enforce and engage with discourses of 'tradition' that are enacted by or centre on women's bodies (Werner 2009; Beyer 2016). But *uyat* is also a discourse of resistance for those who want to question or counter such practices. When a young female blogger discusses her sexual life, or posts her semi-naked or sexualized photos or selfies online and makes these posts public, she directly counters and challenges traditionalizing practices by systematically transgressing expected behaviour.[17] When a self-made exotic dancer from Karaganda covered in tattoos and piercings opened her Instagram account for the public, she, too, resists the *uyat* discourse and attacks it with her own objectification of her sexuality, which she recasts as sexual and bodily liberation. In all these representations, female bodies (or rather ethnicized female bodies) become both a battleground for and a weapon against 'tradition' (see also Beyer and Kojobekova 2019). This is not only a local debate but made possible and exacerbated through tapping into globalized discourses and taking part in online social media.

But if shaming (including on social media) can push one to depression or even suicide,[18] then the focus on bodily liberation and open sexualization aims to counter such practices. It also explains why most active bloggers and those who position themselves as feminist commentators on Instagram in Kazakhstan and Russia focus on the body. It is thus through turning their own private sphere and their own bodies into a 'weapon of the weak' (Scott 1987) that citizens, such as the ones mentioned in this article, have come to target the retraditionalization in the public sphere from above and by authorities. Uyat-man is an example of the power dimension of these discussions, when a non-state actor can enter discussions about 'tradition' with his own interests and his own agenda.

Social media such as Instagram play an important role in shaping norms and perceptions globally but also locally. Instagram most importantly serves as a space for disciplining the visual, the body and the global-local debates on tradition and globalization. Instagram is a space of both visualization and re-creation of new forms of 'acceptable' behaviour and lifestyles locally as well as a site for new globalized perceptions, lifestyles and habits, including sexual liberation and queerness, which lead to local conflicts and resentment online. Complex webs of groups, users and influencers clash over the ultimate meaning of tradition, national identity, gender, sexual practices and essentially what is allowed and not allowed to by exposed visually through the body and bodily lifestyle online. Virtual space rapidly becomes the space for open discussions but also the disciplining area for new practices of traditionalization and activities, such as those carried out by Uyatman in Kazakhstan or Labuten_vsemu_golova in Russia.

Conclusion

Social media greatly shapes local perceptions and values. It influences categories of identification and meaning-making through debates on gender roles, through framing political participation and even by influencing the definition of what counts as 'national tradition'.

Instagram remains a porous and ever-accessible social network that reinforces different views though still serving as a tool for defenders of 'tradition' and global trends alike. Essentially, Instagram destroys these rigid categories and enables a more contextual and diverse understanding of these norms and disciplining practices, even for those who continue to shame others, and it definitely empowers those who aim to resist them. The June 2019 political protests in Russia and Kazakhstan calling for the liberation of journalist Ivan Golunov in Russia,[19] and the June 2019 protests for the fair and open presidential elections in Kazakhstan[20] demonstrated that Instagram can shift from discussions about beauty and tradition to the political realm. This is evident, for example, in the way many civil activists in Russia and Kazakhstan are using Instagram, and other social media such as Facebook and Telegram, to spread information on protests, demands and messages about imprisoned activists online. They usually do so ahead of conventional media reporting, which often remains silent about these protests.[21]

From the livestreams of the protests in Almaty after the 9 June 2019 presidential election, to the Instagram stories of Madina Musina, to the Instagram streams of courtrooms where journalists and activists were being tried in Russia and Kazakhstan, we see that despite the growing authoritarian grip on conventional and new media, these platforms are actively used to transmit all sorts of agendas and messages.

In this study a question remains regarding the power of the content, the power of the online influencer with thousands of virtual followers, commentators and daily viewers, and the power of those who frame the agenda and the message online. Is it the popular power of slut-shaming, calling out ever-changing traditional values, or the power of young women who use their own bodies and their own faces to draw attention to the never-relenting 'my body, my rules' message? In conditions of new global challenges, the popularity of social media, where blocking access to Twitter, WhatsApp, Telegram, Facebook or Instagram demobilizes communities, cities and citizens across the countries of the new hybrid authoritarianism, it is important not to overlook the role social media plays in shaping the diverse discourses of the ever atomizing and compartmentalizing notion of 'communities' within state or social categories. That both Russia and Kazakhstan, along with other undemocratic states, aim to tighten access to social media and control all the multiple online discourses despite the high price of such surveillance and control demonstrates their awareness of the power of social media to channel dissent and alternative voices.[22]

Notes

1. For an interview with Zere Asylbek, see Kate Herrington-Kobekpaeva, 'Run the world: Zeré Asylbek called out gender disparity in Kyrgyzstan and she's only getting started', *Calvert*

Journal, 2 October 2018, https://www.calvertjournal.com/articles/show/10689/zere-asylbek-feminist-pop-anthem-interview (accessed 24 June 2019).
2. For photos and further information see https://www.nur.kz/1072888-vozmutivshuyu-astanchan-statuyu-devushki.html (accessed 10 August 2017).
3. For further details see Aktan Rysaliev, 'Drawing Out Kazakstan's Social Tensions', Institute for War & Peace Reporting, 3 August 2016, https://iwpr.net/global-voices/drawing-out-kazakstans-social-tensions (accessed 5 November 2017).
4. A Pew Research (2016) worldwide survey reported that

> to a greater extent than the other social platforms measured in this survey, Instagram use is especially high among younger adults. Roughly six-in-ten online adults ages 18–29 (59%) use Instagram, nearly double the share among 30- to 49-year-olds (33%) and more than seven times the share among those 65 and older (8%).

Instagram is also a very global social media platform; more than 65% of its users are outside the United States (Highfield and Leaver 2015, 10).
5. Research on social media use in Russia by Russian Search Marketing. Statista's report, 'Leading Countries Based on Number of Instagram Users', places Russia fifth in worldwide Instagram users, with more than 35 million.
6. Data from Amnesty International, 'Think Before You Post: Closing Down Social Media Space in Kazakhstan' (2017) and 2017 NapoleonCat data.
7. In November 2018, Madina Musina had 71,800 followers on Instagram, Diana Idris had 13,600, and Aadya (who had changed her accounts numerous times due to hacks and threats) had more than 20,000.
8. I decided to follow these two publics for a shorter period for two reasons. First, in a year I had collected enough evidence on 'slut-shaming', since both accounts widely shared this type of derogative data. Second, Koten-Insta ceased to exist and Labuten_vsemu_golova stopped posting due to many complaints, which got some of the content deleted almost as soon as it was published. The main editor/s who provided defaming of Instagram female beauty bloggers eventually resigned, and the new editors could not keep the public going or maintain its popularity. I searched and followed these and other similar publics throughout the five-year period, but my main focus remained with the three targeted bloggers mentioned above.
9. Instagram is similar to Twitter in that people need to start 'following' updates from any particular user or public. These followers then can express their appreciation and support by 'liking' any particular post or commenting on any given picture or video that has been shared by the user or the public.
10. The song's lyrics asked the woman whether she earned her luxurious lifestyle, with expensive cars, fur coats and diamonds, via oral sex; a female voice replied, 'No, it was a present.'
11. The deleted blogger's account was traceable at first through her name and came up in the search as 'deleted account' until even her profile was removed from Instagram. Eventually, the editor(s) of Labuten_vsemu_golova were forced to take the video down, but the public was not banned, and they continued to expose other female beauty bloggers and call them sex workers. By the end of my digital ethnography for this project, Labuten_vsemu_golova had lost most of its audience; it was rumoured that the previous editor(s) had left the account, and it soon became less popular and less visible.
12. In February 2018, a public scandal including Russia's deputy prime minister and a famous Russian oligarch developed quickly, creating a precedent of legally obliging Instagram users to delete photos, information and mentions of certain public names from their Instagram accounts. The scandal developed after the leader of the opposition, Alexey Navalny, discovered that the deputy PM and a famous oligarch had travelled together to Norway on a private yacht and discussed politically important matters in the company of sex workers. One of these sex workers, then a popular Russian Instagrammer, Nastya Rybka, published photos, information and even audio and video information from the yacht in her book and widely on her numerous Instagram accounts. I had been following the group related to

Rybka and other 'huntresses' – sexually liberated women who promote free sex and the use of oligarchs (whom they 'hunt') for a year when the scandal broke in the beginning of 2018. Their nude photos, numerous accounts, public sex videos and threats to reveal more information about oligarchs were often deleted, but the story involving the deputy PM and the oligarch finally created a legal precedent in Russia over defamatory and harmful public images of people whose names or pictures are used on Instagram without their consent. Instagram's privacy policy to date has loose ends concerning public damage to one's image or the use of photos. On 25 Feburary 2018, just two weeks after Russia's oppositional leader Alexey Navalny published the video about the oligarch affair with Rybka online, Nastya Rybka and her group were imprisoned in Thailand for providing sexual services. When they were returned to Russia in mid-January 2019, they were briefly imprisoned there. Nastya Rybka, a Belarusian citizen, was released from a Moscow prison at the end of January 2019, when she gave a number of interviews, mainly for YouTube bloggers, but soon after that she disappeared from the popular media.

13. See http://expertonline.kz/a14855/ for a review of the book. http://www.ratel.kz/outlook/opus_mady with book details has been blocked.
14. 'Influencers generally have large social media followings and are assumed to be trusted voices that can reach large audiences' (Carter 2016, 2).
15. Interview with Diana Idris for Buro 24/7 Kazakhstan, http://www.buro247.kz/buro-choise/opinion/diana-idris-eto-bylo-by-smeshno-esli-by-ne-bylo-tak-grustno.html, accessed 10 August 2017.
16. Most of the local LGBTQ bloggers I followed tried to hide their identities and sexuality for security reasons. I also received a number of videos and stories of police abusing LGBTQ people.
17. See also Beyer and Kojobekova in this special issue. For more on the anti-*uyat* campaign, see the recent incident with topless Instagram blogger Shirin Narchayeva in Kazakhstan, "Hundreds of men protest against Shirin Narchayeva's naked photos", https://365info.kz/2019/01/sotni-muzhchin-ustroili-miting-protiv-shirin-narchaevoj/ (accessed 9 January 2019). In winter 2019 a scandal broke out after 18-year-old Shirin Narchaeva posted her topless photos in a *saukele*, the national Kazakh headpiece, on Instagram.
18. In her study of suicides among girls and female teenagers (ages 15–19) in Kazakhstan, Bagayeva (2012) mentions the moral pressures of premarital sex, early pregnancies and immoral behaviour in general as important factors in suicide in Kazakhstan, which is a country that occupies one of the leading places in teenage suicide rates.
19. NBC report on protests in Russia to free Meduza news portal investigative journalist Ivan Golunov: https://www.nbcnews.com/think/opinion/russia-s-decision-free-ivan-golunov-shows-protests-against-kremlin-ncna1018696.
20. Joanna Lillis report on Kazakhstan's protest movements in June 2019: https://eurasianet.org/kazakhstan-waking-up-to-reform.
21. For details on the 'Free Ivan Golunov' protests and how these were discussed on social media, see https://www.rferl.org/a/demonstrators-gather-for-march-to-support-russian-journalist-despite-his-release/29995113.html; and for the Reuters report on Kazakhstan's post-2019 presidential elections protests, also reporting on social media use, see https://uk.reuters.com/article/uk-kazakhstan-election-protests/kazakh-activists-call-for-more-protests-over-presidential-vote-idUKKCN1TC0GA.
22. Netblocks.org has reported that blocking the Internet and various social media in Kazakhstan cost the country more than USD 7 million per hour.

Acknowledgements

I want to thank the guest editors of this special issue, Judith Beyer and Peter Finke, for overseeing and making this collaboration possible. I thank Judith Beyer, Madeleine Reeves and the three anonymous reviewers for their comments, which helped me improve it.

Disclosure statement

No potential conflict of interest was reported by the author.

References

Bagayeva, E. V. 2012. *Devochki Kazakhstana: Pravo na zhizn: analiticheskiy document*. Almaty: Institute of Equal Rights and Equal Opportunities of Kazakhstan. [Kazakhstan's Girls: the right to live: analytical report].

Bamman, D., B. O'Connor, and N. Smith. 2012. "Censorship and Deletion Practices in Chinese Social Media." *First Monday* 17 (3): 3–5. doi:10.5210/fm.v17i3.3943

Beyer, J. 2016. *The Force of Custom: Law and the Ordering of Everyday Life in Kyrgyzstan*. Pittsburgh: Pittsburgh University Press.

Beyer, J., and A. Kojobekova. 2019. "Women of Protest, Men of Applause. Political Activism, Gender and Tradition in Kyrgyzstan." *Central Asian Survey* 38 (3): 329–345. doi:10.1080/02634937.2019.1631258

Beyer, J., and P. Finke. 2019. "Practices of Traditionalization in Central Asia." *Central Asian Survey* 38 (3): 310–328. doi:10.1080/02634937.2019.1636766

Bruns, A., and J. Burgess. 2011. "The Use of Twitter Hashtags in the Formation of ad hoc Publics." In *Proceedings of the 6th European Consortium for Political Research (ECPR) General Conference 2011*, 1–4. Reykjavik: University of Iceland.

Burgess, J., E. Cassidy, S. Duguay, and B. Light. 2016. "Making Digital Cultures of Gender and Sexuality with Social Media." *Social Media + Society* 2 (4): 1–4. doi:10.1177/2056305116672487

Carr, C., and R. Hayes. 2015. "Social Media: Defining, Developing, and Divining." *Atlantic Journal of Communication* 23 (1): 46–65. doi:10.1080/15456870.2015.972282

Carter, D. 2016. "Hustle and Brand: The Sociotechnical Shaping of Influence." *Social Media + Society* 2 (3): 1–12. doi:10.1177/2056305116666305

Castells, M. 2015. *Networks of Outrage and Hope: Social Movements in the Internet Age*. Hoboken, NJ: John Wiley & Sons.

Cirucci, A. 2017. "Normative Interfaces: Affordances, Gender, and Race in Facebook." *Social Media + Society* April-June 2017, 1–10.

Duguay, S. 2016. "Lesbian, Gay, Bisexual, Trans, and Queer Visibility Through Selfies: Comparing Platform Mediators Across Ruby Rose's Instagram and Vine Presence." *Social Media + Society* 2 (2): 1–12. doi:10.1177/2056305116641975

Duffy, B. E., and E. Hund. 2015. ""Having it All" on Social Media: Entrepreneurial Femininity and Self-Branding among Fashion Bloggers,"." *Social Media + Society* 1 (2): 1–11. doi:10.1177/2056305115604337

Featherstone, M., M. Hepworth, and B. S. Turner, eds. 1991. *The Body: Social Process and Cultural Theory*. London: Sage.

Foucault, M. 1990. *The History of Sexuality. Vol. 1: An Introduction*. New York, NY: Vintage Books.

Fournier, V. 2002. "Fleshing Out Gender: Crafting Gender Identity on Women's Bodies." *Body and Society* 8 (2): 55–77. doi:10.1177/1357034X02008002004

Highfield, T., and T. Leaver. 2015. "A Methodology for Mapping Instagram Hashtags." *First Monday* 20 (1): 1–11.

Instagram, Terms of Use. n.d. Accessed August 5, 2017. https://help.instagram.com/478745558852511.

Kirey-Sitnikova, Y. 2016. "The Emergence of Transfeminism in Russia." *TSQ: Transgender Studies Quarterly* 3 (1-2): 165–174. doi:10.1215/23289252-3334343

Kudaibergenova, D. T. 2016. "The Archaeology of Nationalizing Regimes in the Post-Soviet Space." *Problems of Post-Communism* 64 (6): 342–355. doi:10.1080/10758216.2016.1184983

Kudaibergenova, D. T. 2017. "Contemporary Public Art and Nation: Contesting "Tradition" in Post-Socialist Cultures and Societies." *Central Asian Affairs* 4 (4): 305–330. doi:10.1163/22142290-00404001

Kudaibergenova, D. T. 2018. "Project "Kelin": Marriage, Women and Re-Traditionalization in Post-Soviet Kazakhstan." In *Women of Asia: Globalization, Development, and Social Change*, edited by M. Najafizadeh, and L. Lindsay, 379–390. London: Routledge.

Kudaibergenova, D. T. 2019. "Compartmentalized Ideology: Presidential Addresses and Legitimation in Kazakhstan." In *Theorizing Central Asian Politics. The State, Ideology and Power*, edited by R. Isaacs, and A. Frigerio, 145–166. London: Palgrave Macmillan.
Lewis, D. 2016. "Blogging Zhanaozen: Hegemonic Discourse and Authoritarian Resilience in Kazakhstan." *Central Asian Survey* 35 (3): 421–438. doi:10.1080/02634937.2016.1161902
Lupton, D. 2017. "Vitalities and Visceralities: Alternative Body/Food Politics in New Digital Media." In *Alternative Food Politics: From the Margins to the Mainstream*, edited by M. Phillipov, and K. Kirkwood, 1–16. London: Routledge.
Madianou, M. 2016. "Polymedia and Ethnography: Understanding the Social in Social Media." *Social Media + Society* 1: 1–3.
Makarychev, A., and S. Medvedev. 2015. "Biopolitics and Power in Putin's Russia." *Problems of Post-Communism* 62: 45–54. doi:10.1080/10758216.2015.1002340
Mamedov, G. 2016. "The Illusion of the Soviet: Conservative Turn in Kyrgyzstan. The Law on Prohibiting 'Gay Propaganda' and the Soviet Discourse of Homosexuality." In *Queer-Communism eto etika* [Queer Communism is an Aesthetic], edited by O. Shatalova, and G. Mamedov, 63–84. Moscow: Svobodnoe Marxistskoe Izdatelstvo.
Olszanowski, M. 2014. "Feminist Self-Imaging and Instagram: Tactics of Circumventing Sensorship." *Visual Communication Quarterly* 21 (2): 83–95. doi:10.1080/15551393.2014.928154
Pearce, K., and J. Vitak. 2015. "Performing Honor Online: The Affordance of Social Media for Survelliance and Impression Management in an Honor Culture." *New Media and Society* 18 (11): 2595–2612.
Pew Research Center. 2016. "Social Media Update 2016." Accessed August 5, 2017. http://www.pewinternet.org/2016/11/11/social-media-update-2016.
Rodulgina, I. 2016. "Russian Homophobia: The History of Production." *Colta.ru*. Accessed September 15, 2016. http://www.colta.ru/articles/raznoglasiya/12008.
Santarossa, S., and S. Woodruff. 2017. "#SocialMedia: Exploring the Relationship of Social Networking Sites on Body Image, Self-Esteem, and Eating Disorders." *Social Media + Society*, April-June: 1–10.
Scott, J. 1987. *Weapons of the Weak: Everyday Forms of Peasant Resistance*. New Haven, NJ: Yale University Press.
Sheldon, P., and K. Bryant. 2016. "Instagram: Motives for its Use and Relationship to Narcissism and Contextual age." *Computers in Human Behavior* 58: 89–97. doi:10.1016/j.chb.2015.12.059
Shirky, C. 2011. "The Political Power of Social Media. Technology, the Public Sphere, and Political Change." *Foreign Affairs* 90 (1): 28–41.
Stella, F., and N. Nartova. 2016. "Sexual Citizenship, Nationalism and Biopolitics in Putin's Russia." In *Sexuality, Citizenship and Belonging. Trans-National and Intersectional Perspectives*, edited by F. Stella, Y. Taylor, T. Reynolds, and A. Rogers, 24–42. London: Routledge.
Tiidenberg, K. 2015. "Odes to Heteronormativity: Presentations of Femininity in Russian-Speaking Pregnant Women's Instagram Accounts." *International Journal of Communication* 9: 1746–1758.
Turner, B. S. 2008. *The Body and Society: Explorations in Social Theory*. London: Sage.
Underberg, N., and E. Zorn. 2013. *Digital Ethnography: Anthropology, Narrative, and New Media*. Austin: University of Texas Press.
Werner, C. 2009. "Bridal Abduction in Post-Soviet Central Asia: Marking a Shift towards Patriarchy through Local Discourses of Shame and Tradition." *Journal of the Royal Anthropological Institute* 15 (2): 314–331. doi:10.1111/j.1467-9655.2009.01555.x
Young, I. M. 1990. *Throwing Like a Girl and Other Essays in Feminist Philosophy and Social Theory*. Bloomington, IN: Indiana University Press.
Yuval-Davis, N. 1997. *Gender and Nation*. London: Sage.

The veterans' gala: the use of tradition in an industrial labour conflict in contemporary Kazakhstan

Tommaso Trevisani

ABSTRACT

Since its privatization in 1995, Kazakhstan's largest steel mill has been in a restructuring process characterized by workforce reduction, augmented pressure on remaining jobs and labour conflict over wages, work conditions and corporate social responsibility. In 2013, in an attempt to re-establish harmonious relationships with workers, management invited the mill's former labour aristocracy to join a newly established veterans' council, a forum resembling traditional *aksakal* councils, to discuss the company's difficult situation. In the context of a banquet in honour of the veterans, tradition became the contested terrain over which labour and capital struggled to endorse their own visions of the industrial future. As corporate capitalist visions of efficiency and professionalism, ethno-national concerns for harmony and stability, and practices rooted in the Soviet labour legacy clash, tradition is staged by actors as a practice which can either affirm or challenge industrial leadership in a labour conflict.

Introduction

> Good evening! Today, dear veterans, we have gathered you on a great occasion: Kurban-ait. … Different nations celebrate Kurban-ait differently, but the essence of this feast is everywhere the same: It is the great feast of monotheism, the first and greatest feast of humanism. On this day people invite friends and close ones. People who once were enemies become friends. People make peace, make plans for the future. It is a unifying holiday. And we are happy today to have you at this table. (O.T. Kamzabaev, director of labour relations, ArcelorMittal Temirtau, 17 October 2013)[1]

In this opening speech, the director of labour relations at Kazakhstan's largest, former Soviet steel works, also known as Karagandinskiy Metallurgicheskiy Kombinat (Karaganda Iron and Steel Works, colloquially, Karmet), was addressing an audience of former workers, engineers and foreign managers invited to a lavish dinner arranged by the company on the occasion of the Muslim feast of Kurban-ait. The setting was the sumptuous dinner hall of the company-owned Steel Hotel, the most distinguished and expensive venue in Temirtau, a rust-belt town in Kazakhstan's Karaganda Region. Renowned for its Indian cuisine, the hotel is frequented mostly by foreign staff on short-term business trips to the steel plant, or used for corporate events such as this gathering. Invited were some 40 men from all over the steel plant's various shop floors. They were sitting at lavishly loaded banquet tables, the dark suits of many of the elderly adorned with Soviet medals and badges, a reminder that the plant, which nowadays is Indian owned, had been Soviet for more than 30 years.

The celebration took the ritualized form of a *toi* (Kaz.: feast or celebration), with food and spectacle, musical accompaniment, and final blessings by religious dignitaries. Alongside the ritualized division into 'guests' (veterans) and 'hosts' (company managers), carefully moderated speeches were alternately performed by veterans and company managers, followed by toasts and heavy alcoholic drinking. Most veterans were appreciative of this belated recognition in the form of a dinner invitation and of the chance to meet with former colleagues not seen in ages. Also present, from the management's side, were the Indian general director, Mr V.M., accompanied by his personal translator, the Polish human resources (HR) director, Mr A.W., and Mr I.Kh., the Czech chief engineer responsible for the production process. They were the company's most important executives and public personalities in Temirtau. Also on the 'host side' were three young women from the company headquarters, secretaries to some senior manager, who sat at a separate table and came to hand over bags of presents to the veterans and to be available for a dance over the musical intermezzos between speeches. A few journalists, the cameraman of the company-owned local TV channel, and a musical ensemble performing Kazakh and Russian hits and classics completed the picture.

The veterans' gala was a unique event generated by unique circumstances. Convening Soviet veterans, some of whom had worked for up to 50 years in the steel plant and were declared atheists, on the occasion of the religious celebration of Kurban-ait, was unprecedented in Temirtau. Even more exceptional was the reason behind the invitation, namely, to establish a new institution, a veterans' council. Conceived for the task of advising and assisting management in difficult choices ahead, it was inspired on the model of the Kazakh traditional *aksakal* council (council of elders), which was influential in pre-Soviet Central Asian societies (Krader 1963; Bacon 1966; Martin 2001; Beyer 2006). Mr Kamzabaev[2] was the dinner's mastermind, initiator and toastmaster (Rus./Georgian *tamadá*, cf. Mühlfried 2006). Himself of veteran's age, he was the only local, the only Kazakh, and the only one not knowing English among the more powerful foreign management directors attending the event. The veterans' gala and the unconventional idea of establishing a veterans' *aksakal* council were Kamzabaev's personal initiative: a deliberate invention of tradition (Hobsbawm and Ranger 1983), presented, as we shall see, as a measure to overcome an impasse in labour–management relations.

By discussing the veterans' gala, in this article I reflect on the uses of tradition in industrial labour conflict in contemporary Kazakhstan. As connoted by Soviet attitudes and practices, the worlds of heavy industry and tradition are diametrically opposed and, at first glance, unlikely bedfellows. While heavy industry was in many ways seen as the pinnacle of Soviet modernity in 'backward' Central Asia, Soviet prejudice against local cultures and forms of religiosity framed tradition as 'traditionalism', the threatening opposite of socialist modernity (Poliakov 1992). While actively suppressing local forms of traditionalism, Soviet policymakers themselves adopted top-down traditionalisms early on by putting tailored 'traditions' to use in the interest of the state (Grant 1996; Igmen 2012). In the post-Soviet climate of national and cultural re-effervescence, such Soviet-devised traditionalization 'from above' has continued, now in the interest of vigorously nationalizing independent states. At the same time, following a global re-assessment of tradition ('multiple modernities', 'indigenization of modernity'), a new interest in local traditions' liveliness, adaptability and multiplicity has triggered new debates on the nature of 'truth' and authenticity.[3] Essentializing approaches gained salience all over post-Soviet Central Asia, as newly independent states used cultural authenticity and tradition to legitimize post-communist rule and even turning it, as in the case of the Uzbek *mahalla*, the traditional neighbourhood community, into a practical tool of governance (Rasanayagam 2011; Massicard and Trevisani 2003). At the same time, scholars were detecting and deconstructing newly emerging traditions 'from below', by focusing on people's inventiveness and industriousness in their dealings with custom (Beyer 2016), on tradition's 'protean nature' and its capacity to be resurrected in new cultural practices (Levin 1999, 258, 307), and on its inclusive and participatory character, which defies authoritarian leadership models (Dubuisson 2014, 73).

Following this interest in tradition's inner workings, I will focus here on how tradition is put to work in labour conflicts among Kazakhstani steelworkers. Tradition surfaces in this context as a way of claiming authority, as a challenge to (or assertion of) the industrial status quo in the steel plant, and as an act of ambition put forward by cultural entrepreneurs. As we shall see, the veterans' gala was permeated with efforts in 'creative' traditionalization: versatile attempts at making, staging and performing references to tradition for strategic goals. While such traditionalization efforts differ in their source of authority, the use intended and the power of performing actors, the veteran's gala shows how tradition can bring some levelling to the uneven field of labour struggle.

Through the analysis of how different agents of traditionalization – managers and veterans – stage their participation in a ritual performance, this article aims at contributing to regional debates on political performativity (Reeves, Rasanayagam, and Beyer 2014) and notions of virtuous leadership (Liu 2012), and to relate these to post-socialist debates on the morality and authority of management in industrial relations (Ashwin 1999; Rogers 2006; Trevisani 2018). I rely on concepts taken from debates on global labour precarity (Hann and Parry 2018; Munck 2013; Neilson and Rossiter 2008) and post-socialist decline and temporality (Burawoy 2002; Collier 2011; Ringel 2018) to show how pre-Soviet, Soviet and neoliberal heritage is deployed in times of crisis and uncertainty.

While focusing on strategic and antagonistic usages of traditions, I show that the ability to deploy them persuasively must refer to visions and values inscribed in shared cultural and moral registers that raise them above the merely instrumental. Persuasive traditionalizations are, essentially, embedded visions of societal renewal (Liu 2012) that resonate with peoples' lived heritage. Compelling traditionalizations rely on 'pervasive essentialisms' (Herzfeld 1997) – the strategic invoking of notions of past harmony for social actors' specific interests in the present. To be effective, such traditionalizations must be able to 'traverse history' (Sahlins 1999, 409) and reach out to meanings, associations and values that are shared, believed and felt collectively. Therefore, an attentive look at the practice of staging and performing tradition must depart from a narrow 'Hobsbawmian' reading of traditionalization, understood as a mere strategic and instrumental manipulation of tradition. When deployed to achieve legitimacy and social consensus in a labour conflict, invoked tradition always conveys underlying concepts of the good and the rightful in industrial relations.

The traditionalization efforts I observe in the veterans' gala raise fundamental questions about the nature of the capitalist project. What should the company be accountable for? Should the steel plant be run as a social enterprise or as economic business? We shall see how such questions emerge from the tensions and frictions underlying the different visions and understandings that motivate the actors of traditionalization. The social responsibility of the society-producing factory; the corporate logic of capitalist profit; the dominant, state-mandated attempt to accommodate industrial identity to newly defined ethnocultural ('nationality') demands: surfacing all over the dinner's heated conversations, such issues mark the divided heritages and visions of the industrial future in steel-town Temirtau. They represent the background against which the traditionalization practices observed in the veteran's gala must be analysed and interpreted.

This article is part of an ethnographic project based on fieldwork carried out in the Temirtau steel plant. At the intersection of global capital, Soviet industrial legacies and Kazakhstani nation-building, it is concerned with changing labour relations, emerging forms of inequality and distinctive patterns of precarity among multi-ethnic steelworkers (Trevisani 2015, 2016, 2018). While the overall project's focus is on shop floor interactions among workers, here I am concerned with how tradition becomes a tool in labour conflict. It is based on the analysis of the veterans' gala, during which, besides those of the four executive directors who were present at the event, I recorded 14 veterans' speeches over the three-hour dinner. By analysing the ritual performance and content of the speeches, the article investigates the different ways local and foreign actors, veterans and management of the steel plant came to understand and tried to impact their industrial present and future by performing tradition.

Protracted stagnation

Temirtau was originally a peasant settlement named Samarkandsky and later part of the Karaganda Gulag (Barnes 2011; Dulatbekov 2012). After the war, it became a mono-industrial town thanks to the construction of its giant steel works. Moulded by Soviet industrial work and development, the mono-industrial town developed a strong community around the Soviet symbiosis of society and factory (Buttino 2015). During the Soviet Union, Karmet was a symbol of socialist modernity.[4] The Soviet plant was technologically up to date and an elite training centre for scientific and political cadres. Many party officials, some of them still renowned and politically active today, have their background in this plant, and today the steel mill is still associated with the president of Kazakhstan, who began his career there as a blast furnace operator.

With the collapse of the Soviet Union the steel plant fell into crisis. Production had nearly stopped and Temirtau's population was rapidly declining, when in 1995 the British-based Indian billionaire Lakshmi Mittal took over the plant from state ownership. Under Mittal's foreign managers, arrears were paid and production gradually recovered with a modicum of investment into the (by then decrepit) machinery. The decline was reversed, and Temirtauians hailed Mittal as a saviour, everyone being aware that 'if the *kombinat* doesn't work, the city will stop existing' (Y.F., veteran).

> You came to us when it had been very hard for us, when our government was in trouble. Thanks to you the city still exists, the city blossoms. As we say, by God, your enterprise – our enterprise. The factory works, we also live very well. (E.T., veteran)

This speech was by a veteran who had worked in the blast furnaces with President Nazarbayev back in the early days of the *kombinat*, and who therefore was often seen at formal corporate meetings and public occasions to perform the role of the president's friend. Addressed to the imaginary presence of Mittal himself, the speech had a reverential tone. It was politely centred around gratitude to and optimism for the company and the government, a message often amplified in official discourses – but in which the complexities and the more contradictory feelings that circulate in Temirtau around Mittal's ownership of the Soviet-built plant remained concealed.

Temirtauians often credited Mittal for mastering the challenge of averting Karmet's foreclosure. By enduring and overcoming difficulties Mittal successfully managed to adapt management to local constraints and conditions. Tax holidays and regulatory exemptions that were part of the undisclosed privatization deal helped keep the plant afloat and eventually, also thanks to the bullish steel conjuncture of the late 1990s and early 2000s, to run it profitably. But after the honeymoon, voices critical of the foreign ownership intensified. Over the years of economic recovery Temirtauians became resentful of 'the Indians' for siphoning away the profits from a factory formerly owned by the people without 'giving back' enough to the city. Accusations were directed against the company's radical job cuts, worsening labour conditions, neglect of environmental issues and non-transparent finances. Since Mittal's arrival, workers have lamented a lack of investment and what many see as exaggerated, 'furious' cost-saving job cuts in the steel plant's many departments and shop floors. Foreign management presented them as inevitable restructuring, necessary to improve profitability and to ensure an economically viable future for the steel works. Workers held the opposite view, fearing that restructuring was undermining the very viability of the steel plant's future. Such worries were echoed in the veterans' speeches:

> Of course, the number of workers had to be reduced, but only to a sustainable degree. In the city, there are many who need to work somewhere, and at the steel plant they are not hiring. The Institute [Temirtau's higher education institute for education and training in metallurgical professions] ... we celebrated its 50th anniversary. The lecture halls were empty. No registrations, even when scholarships are available! If registration numbers fall, this is because students getting their degrees from that institute end up working in the bazaar. (Y.F., veteran)

Worries about the loss of intergenerational knowledge transmission were expressed, and demands for jobs to be transferred across generations were put forward, since these chains of knowledge and skills passed on through families were being interrupted nowadays, because of company jobs no longer being available in the plant. The same veteran quoted above drew attention to the double drama of job scarcity in the city and worker scarcity on the shop floor. To him, it would be 'better to pay a smaller salary, but employ more people', a philosophy strongly opposed by the current management.

By the time of my fieldwork, the steel plant was again navigating troubled waters. Problems in production, procurement, supply and marketing had worsened. With market competition growing and prices falling, labour–management relations had gradually become more confrontational. After the end of the Soviet Union Temirtau had become more socially divided as a consequence of privatization, restructuring and nation-building. The Soviet stratification has been thoroughly shaken in the post-Soviet period as result of political-economic transformations and migratory flows. Social divides have opened up between regular and precarious workers, between 'townspeople' and 'factory people',[5] and between groups of different ethnicities, such as culturally 'Russian' (Slavic or

Russianized non-Slavic) long-term residents, who still constitute the majority in Temirtau, and newly arrived Kazakhs, the growing minority. By and large everyday relations are unproblematic and peaceful, as proclaimed in the post-Soviet Kazakhstani ideology of multi-ethnic harmony, which stands for ethnic tolerance and pluralism in a multi-ethnic state. However, as elsewhere in Kazakhstan (cf. Moscaritolo 2012), resentments linger. Predominantly Russian steelworkers are often sceptical of an independence which they see as prioritizing Kazakh interests over theirs. Speaking publicly about these problems is taboo, yet many better-skilled Russian workers have found employment elsewhere and left the country. Despite growing differences, the 'Indians' had the merit of unifying an increasingly divided town around joint criticism of the foreign ownership and management.

We see that Temirtau's working people reside in a context of crisis and restructuring similar to that known from industrial settings affected by post-socialist decline and shrinking (Ringel 2018; Burawoy 2002; Mrozowicki 2011), with the difference that, rather than steep decline and deindustrialization, Temirtau's industrial trajectory faces a more gradual decay and protracted stagnation. Elsewhere, I have termed this oblique downward trajectory, captured neither by post-industrial shrinkage nor by post-post-socialist recovery, a 'partial intensification' of the industrial regime (Trevisani 2018, 105). In this context, capital is reluctant to invest in radical restructuring (arguably fearing government interference), thus maintaining labour employed under deteriorating shop floor conditions. The government accepts this compromise because it limits the erosion of jobs and industrial welfare, while labour suffers worsening health and safety conditions and has to make up for the production shortcomings caused by ageing machines and lack of investment (Kesküla 2018).

In Temirtau's post-privatization trajectory, workers and the city feel trapped by the 'presentism' (Guyer 2007; Ringel 2018) of the precarious balance that keeps the factory running, at the same time remaining sceptical of management's and the government's respective promises of a radiant future. Workers, as elsewhere under flexible labour regimes, are facing devaluation and precarization of their labour and a crisis in the meaning and ethos of their work (cf. Rajković 2017). Still, under the particular constellation of capital, labour and the encompassing Kazakhstani state, workers in Temirtau are not giving up on their visions and values and hard work, thanks to which the plant, and the city, continue to cope and survive. Steel has lost its former Soviet glory, but it continues to define the city's core identity and economy.

The authoritarian state takes an ambiguous stance between capital and labour, by preempting both real criticism and a thorough reform of the employment regime. It thus contributes to shaping a form of balanced stagnation, in which company managers' and workers' expectations and understandings of each other's entitlements and roles never meet. 'Russian' workers idealize the Soviet past and develop, in workers' parlance, a *chemodannoe nastroienie* (lit., 'mood for packing suitcases': a desire to leave the country at the first opportunity), while Kazakh workers look more hopefully at the national future, even as their prospects for social mobility promise to be post-industrial ones. At the same time, corporate foreigners are frustrated by their inability to implement thoroughly 'efficient' (read: neoliberal) labour restructuring. In such a context, low-intensity labour conflict has become the new normal, also because trade unionism and effective collective action is tolerated by the government only up to a certain point.[6] While Soviet workers enjoyed the system's promise of a 'normal life' (Yurchak 2006, 118–9) – dignified work, social welfare and an inclusive workplace sociality – dissatisfied post-Soviet workers complain about the company, voice anger at work, and work recalcitrantly, but are sceptical about their own ability to articulate more effective resistance to the new corporate labour regime.

Tools in labour conflict

In 2013, the causes of the factory's crisis had become the object of heated debate between management and the trade union. Workers lamented the harsh working conditions and the decay of the ageing factory. For management, the company was losing market share because of the high costs and poor quality of production. The trade union accused the company of taking advantage of crisis talks to justify unnecessary austerity measures. While only some of the company workers backed the trade union in their criticism (the others arguing that it wasn't going far enough), all agreed that the factory's difficult moment necessitated action and lamented the poor working conditions.

The directors of HR and labour relations, Mr A.W. and Mr Kamzabaev, took an active role in the negotiation with the trade union, but over time they found themselves in growing disagreement, the one pushing for more job cuts, the other vehemently opposing them. Kamzabaev's sympathies were, he said, for the 'people' and for the 'factory', not for the trade unions. Equally critical of the 'Indians' and the local shop floor managers, he saw in management both the factory's problem and the key to reform. His plea for management renewal was informed by his philosophy of the three P's: *professionalizm, patriotizm,* and *poriyadochnost'* (decency). *Flow*, a book by Chicago organizational psychologist Csikszentmihalyi (1990), was his favourite reference. During our conversations, the pictures on his office wall of quality control expert W. Edwards Deming, British naval historian Cyril Northcote Parkinson and Soviet telepathist Wolf Messing were points of departure for many a digression on his ideas about good management.

With negotiations for the collective labour agreement having reached a deadlock and under the urgency of the plant's economic difficulties, Mr Kamzabaev came up with an attempt at 'inventing' a tradition, by calling for a meeting of the steel plant's veterans. In a broader sense, the event was an experiment aimed at winning the favour of what, in the eyes of management, was the influential group of the former labour aristocracy (elite workers and shop floor managers).[7]

In Temirtau, steel veterans are a reputable influence group. Although they are not organized into an association, many are well connected and follow the vicissitudes of the steel plant; after retirement they still feel concerned because of their family linkages or other interest in their former place of employment. No census exists, but invited veterans themselves estimated their number in the hundreds or even around a thousand. By approaching a limited number of particularly reputable individuals, Mr Kamzabaev wanted to involve this group of stakeholders in his efforts to mitigate public suspicion of Mittal, by convincing veterans to give their public support in a difficult moment for the company. Although veterans do not exert direct influence over the trade union, the symbolic significance of their consent was deemed worth pursuing by Mr Kamzabaev.

Mr Kamzabaev prepared the event carefully over several weeks, compiling lists of veterans and holding informal talks. After public talks over the renewal of labour agreements between trade union and management had ended in open quarrelling and bad press, inviting veterans and honouring Kurban-ait seemed to promise better headlines for the company: it appeared to be a welcome initiative both for the Kazakhs, who saw Kurban-ait as one of their national celebrations so far disregarded in the company's PR, and for the 'Russian' workers, who knew about Soviet celebrations for labour veterans, later discontinued after privatization.

Mr Kamzabaev himself was a newcomer to the steel department. Trained as a retail manager, he had worked in the Soviet years in various state-owned companies and lastly in the coal mining department of ArcelorMittal in Karaganda. There he stayed until recently, when the company moved its headquarters to Temirtau. The son of a renowned family of academics, he grew up outside the world of industry. Equally close to (or distant from) the working people of Temirtau, the company management he criticized and cherished, and the Kazakh state, whose closest representative he was in the foreign-dominated top management, Kamzabaev's role in the plant came closest to that of a company intellectual. Such characters are no strangers to large corporate enterprises, which rely on local intellectual and cultural resources when it comes to justifying and vernacularizing neoliberal restructuring policies into local idioms of inequality (Sanchez 2012). But Kamzabaev's case goes in the opposite direction: banking on Soviet and Kazakh heritage, he challenges corporate conduct from the inside, by engaging tradition and its implicit values to rein in a dispute with labour. Over various initiatives that he had organized to promote 'labour harmony' between workers and management, he became critical of management, especially of the HR director, whom he likened to a 'bad gardener' (*plokhoi sadovnik*) for his indiscriminate cuts and spending reviews. The difference in views gradually turned into antagonism, as the two directors found themselves holding diametrically opposed views on the future of the plant and how to implement restructuring. The foreign HR manager's job was to implement cuts, but the local manager was vehemently opposed to them and accused the former of undermining the plant's prospects by not appropriately valuing its staff. Despite the diplomatic tone of their speeches, the acrimony between the two was hardly concealed during the gala. Although the union talks were not explicitly mentioned (not inviting trade unions or state representatives was part of Kamzabaev's effort to keep the tone of the talks within the harmonious framework of a feast and to avoid putting embarrassing quarrels on public display), those attending the dinner were all aware of the latent tensions setting the 'town' in opposition to 'Indians', and locals against foreigners.

Mr Kamzabaev was hoping that the veterans' dinner would help win the support of the Indian general director, to overcome the HR director's 'blockade' of the talks with the trade unions. While his general aim was to establish labour harmony in the interest of the company, his personal interest was to demonstrate managerial skills and thus boost his career.

> These aren't just people sitting here, but experienced professionals, people who have seen life, who have passed on their knowledge to their children. … As we used to say, we have labour dynasties [*trudovye dinastii*], and members of our dynasties are here with us today: their children work with us, now they are managers in our company. (Kamzabaev)

Kamzabaev's pledge not to waste their experience went down well with the veterans, who felt emboldened and thankful for this recognition. His speech, and the gala in general, were well received by the veterans, because they were so different from the conventional corporate PR they were used to. Although the dinner's ceremonial form followed the corporate style, which mixes Soviet, Kazakh and Indian elements into a single form, in other respects the event was very different from conventional corporate events, particularly in invoking tradition and using it as a tool in labour negotiations. By referencing Kazakh *aksakaldar* (elders) and 'Soviet veterans', tradition was put to work to legitimize a new institution that promised to embody positive aspects of both the Soviet and the Kazakh past. But unlike the socially palliative and politically correct corporate PR, the veterans' gala was envisioned as a new tradition with the capacity to challenge the social and political status quo.

Corporate traditionalization

As elsewhere in Central Asia, Soviet ceremonial practice and public celebrations have been redefined in Kazakhstan since independence (Adams 2010; Roy 1997; Laruelle 2007). The independent state has valorized ethnic nationhood, but maintained significant continuity with Soviet practice when it comes to cultural forms, rites and styles of celebration. Within Karmet, Soviet rites, symbolic hierarchies (such as the wall of honour (*pochetnaya doska*) for the best workers of the month, prizes and rewards for the best brigade, etc.), feasting and celebrations that were an integral part of work and life in the Soviet Union have survived privatization in modified form. This continuity is reinforced by the fact that, to forestall local criticism, only a very few foreign top managers have been sent to Temirtau since privatization, the bulk of staff still consisting of the local workforce and labour dynasties that were 'raised' in the Soviet plant. Although celebrations with veterans were common in the past, after privatization, Soviet labour celebrations were downsized under the post-privatization corporate spending review or replaced by new public celebrations with different symbolic connotations, while those for Karmet's veterans were discontinued altogether. Outside the steel plant, the company organizes public events and participates in the calendar of public celebrations, for instance by setting up corporate yurts and sponsoring concerts for the Nauryz holiday, the Central Asian New Year celebrated in March, as the government and the city expects it to do. On the first of May, which is no longer a workers' holiday but now the (multi)national Day of Unity of the People of Kazakhstan, the company organizes marches and concerts, as it does for International Women's Day, New Year's Day and other national holidays. During public concerts and marches, such as the traditional Steelworkers' Day in July, pictures of Mittal and the president shaking hands are displayed in tabloids, while Indian songs and dances are now included in the multinational folklore and musical entertainment put on stage for festive occasions. The new corporate ceremonial culture thus adopts Soviet cultural forms that make it recognizable and appreciated, since they resonate with local experience and expectations. Although they are at odds with modern corporate management culture, the company deemed it important to maintain rites and celebrations and preserved them in modified form, with an eye to balancing costs and benefits. Celebrations like that for Women's day or the Nauryz concert are now smaller but more elegant and glamorous, performed in a way better suited for television. Workers charge that in the past these were larger, more inclusive events.

In the eyes of many workers, corporate spending on these kinds of public celebrations and philanthropy is 'hollow' and 'insincere', since the foreign company has come 'for the profit, not for the good of the people' (M.Yu., steelworker). The Soviet plant was an all-enveloping provider of housing, heating, food, education, health, recreation and other services to its employees and to the city (cf. Collier 2011). The privatized steel plant has not followed up on the Soviet plant's all-encompassing care, but it does engage in some philanthropic activity in the framework of its corporate social responsibility policy. It sponsors scholarships at local high schools, maintains sports facilities for its employees, subsidizes public transport and runs a clinic for its employees. Still, many dissatisfied workers accuse the company of greed and stinginess. They resent the foreign ownership of the steel plant and dismiss corporate philanthropy as a waste of money that would be better spent on hiring more workers.

Corporate philanthropy backfires, paradoxically ending up only reinforcing workers' hostility and prejudice, despite the company's efforts to draw from the accepted repertoire of Soviet and national cultural forms and ritual legacies for its PR and corporate social responsibility campaigns. The company is aware of this, which might also be one reason it prioritizes investment in the media and public visibility rather than ceremonial expenditures, deeming the first rational, since it promises to increase acceptance and quiescence among dissatisfied and often hostile workers, and the second only a necessary burden, rooted in expectations shaped by the Soviet legacy that can never be met. Thus, the elaborate PR and corporate social spending helps contain criticism, with corporate-owned local media promulgating a positive public image of the privatized plant. All the same, these attempts at claiming local traditions for corporate PR are met with suspicion locally.

The conventional corporate PR pattern conflating corporate culture with local traditions repeated itself in the general director's and HR's performances at the veterans' gala. Kamzabaev's speech was followed by that of the general director.

> Good evening, veterans. I would like to wish you all in Arabic, *Ait mubarak*. Which is Kurban-ait. Basically, as you know, this is to honour people who sacrifice. I'm personally standing here thanks to your hard work. I also thank you for training your children, your grandchildren, who are all working here. Today, the current team is full of challenges because of the market. The interior team is focused on bringing the plant back to its original glory. You will also personally see that from your relatives working in the plant, how focused we all are on this. And from this year on, we would like to meet all of you every six months. And I also would like to receive your feedback on how we can do better. Be free to give your suggestions so that we can change, because you have seen good and bad in the past. *Spasibo* [Thank you]. (General Director V.M.)

The Indian general director's speech addressed the two reasons for the ceremony: the Muslim feast and the veterans' gathering. It also gave performative fiat to the veteran's council, by stating that the institution would come together regularly from now on. In his speech, the general director claimed religious competence by trying to make use of religious repertoire (his good wish in Arabic and his reference to sacrifice as the central meaning of Kurban-ait), and acknowledged the veterans' 'sacrifice', their merits, and Karmet's Soviet 'glory'. He blamed 'the market' for the current challenges, and praised the workers' 'focus'. By making the rounds of all the tables and greeting every single veteran with a handshake, he expressed humility, but also leadership and presence. However, the invitation to speak out, on the guarantee that their advice would be taken seriously, was contradicted by the fact that he and the HR director, the factory's number two, left the meeting immediately after having greeted all the veterans, citing 'other business'. In doing so, they again created distance and hierarchy between themselves and the veterans.

At the gala, the general director, the only one wearing the blue company work uniform at the dinner, performed his closeness to the 'factory people' to overcome their distance and diffidence. But he also performed power and hierarchy, in affirming his leadership over the plant and over Kamzabaev's potentially insubordinate initiative. Unlike Kamzabaev's, his performance was an attempt at a traditionalization practice cementing the status quo of power relations, made by staging rituals that hinted at local cultural forms but that also performatively enacted power discrepancies, leadership and hierarchy. Veterans noticed the contrast between management's 'nice words' and its deeds, essentially finding their prejudice and diffidence against the foreigners reconfirmed.

Whereas Mr Kamzabaev and the general director centred their rhetorical efforts on the acknowledgement of the veterans, in his speech the HR director focused on the Polish-Kazakh history and on the importance of paying respect to the elders. In a short speech that was received coolly by the veterans, the HR director, who was at the centre of criticism for being in charge of implementing job cuts, focused on the past and present of Polish–Kazakh friendship, in the style of the Soviet trope of *druzhba narodov* (Friendship of Peoples), but omitting the underlying problems and trying to justify his foreignness. 'Kazakhstani steelworkers are being hired by ArcelorMittal in Poland', he told the veterans, '[so] do not mind if one Polish manager is working in Kazakhstan.' By avoiding the mention of job cuts and the purpose of the gala, he disenfranchised the initiative of his competitor, Kamzabaev. The reference to eldership was ambiguous: it could be read as meaning 'don't waste your time on politics, stay with your families'; or as 'respect the management, your "elder brother"' – that is, if you criticize, you will not go far – subtly evoking memories of the Zhanaozen 2011 event, a labour protest that was cracked down on by the government, as was well known to everyone in the factory. Like the general director, he left immediately after his speech, citing another meeting. The veterans would spend the rest of the dinner giving speeches to the absent general director and HR director, the factory's two top managers. The Czech chief engineer (whose short talk focused on reporting the state of progress of the modernization of the plant by rattling off the millions in investment for projects executed or planned) and Mr Kamzabaev would be the only two directors listening to the veterans for the rest of the celebration.

The veterans

> Dear metallurgists, it is a great feast for us today. Each of us worked in this plant for no less than 40 years. We've spent our youth, our life in this place. We honestly worked hard and deservedly went off to rest. (E.T., veteran)

To the veterans, the meeting was as much an occasion for addressing their concerns to company representatives as it was for commemoration, to celebrate their common history, and to remember those who had passed away. Although gathered on the pretext of establishing an advisory body, re-evoking an emotionally loaded past in the factory was also important and resounded with veterans' experiences, with their expectations of moral commitment and status shaped over the Soviet period (Edele 2008).

While the veterans' foremost reason for joining the gala lay in their concern for the future of the steel plant, the evening was also a welcome occasion to perform their 'veteran-ness': staging their role as veterans and speaking publicly about their experience in the Soviet plant. As Y.F., a veteran, said: 'I'm saying "our" [factory], because we came out of it. Also, right now, someone [we have trained] is working there. For this reason, the factory is, essentially, ours.'

In their speeches, veterans acknowledged their strong attachment to the steel plant; a recurring phrase was *rodnoi kombinat* (native plant). Karmet was likened to a homeland, because 'we came out if it', 'we worked there', 'we built it', and 'those trained by us still work there'. In Soviet years, nearly every adult in Temirtau was directly or indirectly on its payroll. The Soviet steel works was the city's central employer and a provider of welfare, housing, education, employment and sociality. Over the Soviet period, steelworkers' families were employed in the plant over several generations, parents preparing their children for work in the plant and priding themselves in transmitting knowledge and status to their offspring (Kesküla 2018). The factory was part of their enculturation and socialization; growing up in Temirtau entailed much of what it took to become an accomplished steelworker later on (cf. Willis 1977). To a lesser degree this still applies today, and therefore, unsurprisingly, at the dinner the veterans expressed deep attachment to a workplace that had shaped their lives and had produced not only steel but also valuable cadres, skilled people with strong character, and industrial elites such as those who now ruled their country, their region and their city. In their speeches, pride and emotional involvement were palpable:

> The plant is a unique industry. In the Soviet Union, we built it with help from all over the Union republics. It is still working now. I think there is a bright future for this plant. Like a living organism, it had peaks and troughs. In 1988 we produced more than five million tons of steel. ... All of us here today had their part in the development of the plant. I wish you all health, happiness, happiness with your grandchildren. (E.T., veteran)

In another speech, by a former worker who had spent his life at the blast furnace (*domna pech*), the factory was also equated to a living organism. In the workers' parlance, each of the four furnaces had a name. This one referred to the furnace's head of workers, a man named Ivanov. The furnace was thus personalized as Donna Ivanovna, portrayed as a complex machine with a history, moods, and a character. Donna Ivanovna was a capricious woman with a soul, who also demanded one's soul and love and dedication if she was to work properly.

Muehlebach (2017) encounters similar organicist tropes and workers' expressions of 'love for machines' and analyses them as traces of a materially grounded community, in which machines produce 'thick social relations' (120), solidarity and values, so strong that they outlive the factory. In similar vein, veterans can claim for themselves and for the other workers a 'thick' moral ownership of their workplace, a source of authority that the real, more powerful, owners lack. This moral authority grounds the veterans' vision of industrial renewal. It structures their claimed entitlement to express criticism and care for the factory.

By highlighting workers' decisive role in the survival of the factory, veterans stress the role of local expertise and its intergenerational transmission to counter the effects of transnationalization on the value of local skills. Veterans not only defend a specific claim to the factory's past, but also narrate the past to counter the transnationalization of expertise and its devaluative effects on local labour. Unlike the company's merely folklorizing use of tradition, veterans invoke an idea of heritage that is vital and essential to the factory's survival, that is part of the factory's 'living tradition' (Sahlins 1999).

The veterans' visions of good management drew from different repertoires, but all were rooted in local traditions and labour legacies, and were articulated in polemics against the foreign management. They expressed anguish at the existential threats to their factory, to workers and their families, and did not hold back from criticizing the management for their shortcomings and responsibilities.

> Let's drink, as our general director said, to dreams. May they become true, may the steel plant thrive again! May it be as before, with no economic, so to speak, crises around. They shall not affect our work! They should not influence it at all, if you are being good managers. ... We, for our part, we'll spill the metal, this, and all the rest, no worries. But you look, look for those holes [in the budget], stop them, stuff them all! Sell! You are the businessmen! (N.N., veteran)

Peculiar class theories were put forward by another veteran, who stated that after the *razval* (the post-socialist breakdown) three classes had emerged: the high, the middle and the working class. The plant's present problems are rooted in the lack of consensus, agreement (*soglasie*), among them. To him, the company's first priority was to re-establish harmony across the classes. In this constellation, the *nachal'niki* (shop floor heads) were portrayed as those who solve problems at the production level, a 'middle class' who make common cause with the workers against 'those above', i.e. the foreign managers. Heckling by other veterans dismissed this class-talk as backward-looking and confused, but the focus of criticism on foreign management again suspended divisions and projected unity.

The veterans' criticism and their proposed remedies for Karmet's problems centred on their vision of good management, a vision different from that of the foreign management and surprisingly coherent across different speeches. It centred around the model of a just and benevolent master (*khoziain*), the paternalistic director of the Soviet era, who saw the workplace as a household, and the workers as his family (Trevisani and Kesküla 2016; Ashwin 1999; Rogers 2006).

> Let the shop floor manager be the master in his own shop. Here sit people who bore the role of shop floor manager on their shoulders. And they know: labour discipline, production, economy – everything was on them. The shop floor manager [*nachal'nik*] mastered all these things. He was the boss in the shop, the master [*khoziain*] of the shop. Let him be the master in his shop and you will be rewarded! (Kh.U., veteran)

Among the veterans, the idea of the shop floor manager as a patriarchal provider and fatherly authority who knows everything about production seemed deeply internalized, and was positioned as the solution to the company's present problems. He was seen as a moral and professional authority (the shop floor's 'master', or even 'draft horse', in one of the veterans' speeches), whose absence had left a void in the post-Soviet shop floor.

The veterans' plea was to reinstall this local model of authority. 'I., please!' said a veteran, heartily addressing the Czech chief engineer by his first name, 'Let the *nachal'nik* be the real master of the shop floor and you will be rewarded. Do not obstruct their work, be supportive, don't change them too frequently.'[8] 'Revitalize the Soviet way of working, empower the *nachal'niki*.'

The veterans' diagnosis of and proposed remedy for the ills of their plant was in direct contradiction to the plans of the foreign management to shrink the role of the once all-powerful *nachal'niki* and to reorganize the working of the shop floor, bypassing them. They refused to acknowledge management's concealed but implicit argument that the factory's poor economic performance today, and the factory's bad shape prior to privatization, could be imputed to the persistence of the Soviet *khoziain* model, or, in other words, to *them*. What the former saw as the solution, the latter saw as Karmet's problem.

Local and corporate paternalisms differ in that they draw from different sources of authority and use tradition in different ways and for different ends. Veterans counter the corporate paternalism in the CEO and HR directors' performance of hierarchy and leadership with local visions grounded in traditions they can reclaim by virtue of their long work in the plant. Veterans reverse the corporate hierarchy by speaking about Soviet legacies (*khoziain* and *nachal'nik*) to which they feel entitled by their sense of moral hold over the factory, staging counter-paternalism 'from below' (Figure 1).

The uses of tradition and its limit

> Dear comrades, I ask the Almighty to hear what was said by the representatives of the previous generation of metallurgists. May the Almighty assist our leaders, first of all the leaders of ArcelorMittal Temirtau. So that ArcelorMittal Temirtau might prosper, thanks to the veterans, and to the workers. I wish you all health and happiness! If we are with Allah, if we carry him always in our souls, we will be healthy and happy. May ArcelorMittal, our city and our homeland, be blessed and prosper. *Allah akbar!* (A.A., veteran)

The veterans' corporate Kurban-ait gala ended with a prayer by a 'veteran-*aksakal*', first in Kazakh, then translated into Russian. Most of the veterans joined him in raising their hands for the ritual gesture *amin*, performed at the end of the prayer. A photo session, the

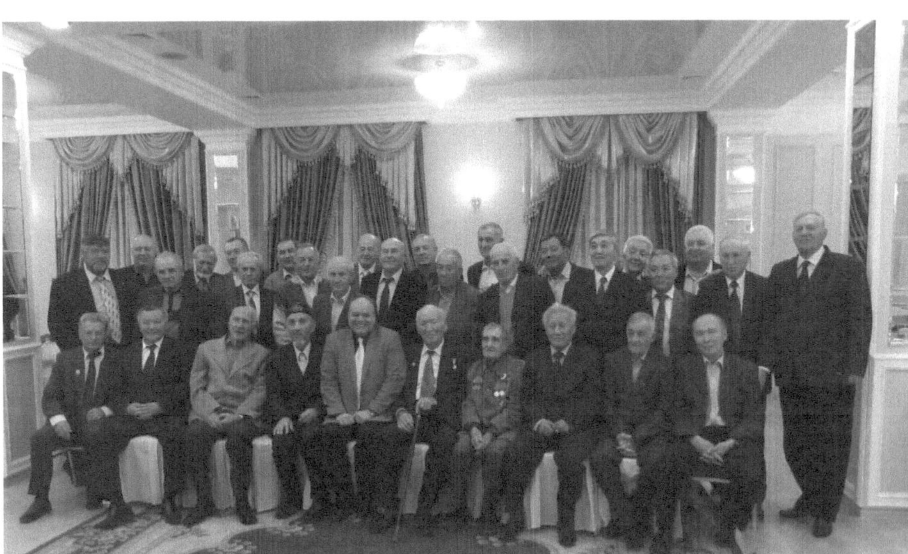

Figure 1. The veteran's dinner at ArcelorMittal Temirtau, 17 October 2013. Photograph by the author.

distribution of gifts, handshakes and farewell chats prolonged the dinner a little longer, before everyone dispersed.

The gala was a unique event brought about by extraordinary circumstances, and must be seen in light of different factors: the labour–management conflict at Temirtau's steel plant; internecine management struggles between local and foreign managers within the company; and the particular framework of ArcelorMittal's PR, which has appropriated and blended Soviet social policies with Kazakhstani national cultural forms and incorporated them into corporate practices. While the foreign management wanted to appease the veterans and downsize the labour force, the local management and the veterans wanted to maintain labour and change the foreign management policy. The veterans' claim came out of a sense of moral ownership that veterans and workers held by virtue of their long years of work in the plant (Trevisani 2018).

Reflecting on the different references, uses, and creative engagements with tradition, the gala shows that despite mutual invocations of harmony, veterans' and management's different understandings of industrial legacies and tradition did not harmonize. Although on the surface they claimed to aim at mutual harmony, in substance they talked at cross-purposes. The lived experience underlying the veterans' sense of tradition, and their pledge for how to revitalize it, was at odds with the company's essentializing attempts to win local support by staging 'Kazakh' and 'Soviet' rituals of recognition, which sounded hollow in workers' ears. The company executives were nominally committed to a politically correct doctrine of multi-ethnic harmony, but felt they had justify their 'foreignness' *vis-à-vis* resentful locals. By turning veterans into *aksakals*, they tapped into a cultural model that resonated with specifically Kazakh forms of tradition and led to the folklorization of a PR-event that could be broadcast on TV. But the veterans did not feel taken seriously by management, despite the solemn declarations of the general director, who then quickly left. After the meeting, managers and veterans were reconfirmed in their irreconcilable differences of views, priorities and values.

In the months after the veterans' gala, Mr Kamzabaev stepped up criticism of the management but did not attempt to revive the *aksakal* council. Eventually he left the company, with no farewell ceremony and in disagreement with management. A regular *aksakal* council was not established in the company, and the veteran's gala remained a unique event, though other feasts and the sponsoring of social and cultural activities continue to be used by management as a palliative to persistent problems and conflicts. Soon, a new cohort of foreign managers, sent from the corporate headquarters, would succeed the generation who took part in the veterans' gala: they will continue to deal with local 'tradition' according to the principles of their corporate PR, no longer having to worry about Mr Kamzabaev's creative attempts to employ it in novel ways and arenas.[9]

Traditionalization recurred in this context as a strategic practice aimed at renegotiating power relations by referring to the authority of tradition. Corporate traditionalization can be seen as an instrument to legitimize and strengthen the corporate grip on an industrial community by stepping into the footprint of local, top-down legacies of 'tradition'. The veteran's gala shows that such an approach can backfire when it fails to persuade those for whom it is intended. For those who lack power but 'have' tradition, tradition can become a 'weapon of the weak' (Scott 1985) in labour conflict, when it is grounded in legacies and values that resonate with peoples' lived experience. In such cases, traditionalization can be a form of ersatz collective action 'from below', effective in countering corporate encroachments while expressing a voice that cannot be simply ignored by powerful foreign managers.

Following Hobsbawm and Ranger's (1983) analysis of how tradition is produced, we can distinguish between a reinvention of tradition from 'above' (i.e. the company, the state policy of public ceremonials) and from 'below' (the veterans' Kurban-ait), which is the case when social actors take up rites and wrap them up in the vestiges of tradition to state their (political) identity in the present, as the local manager did. In both cases, traditionalization surfaces as a tool in the struggle for meaning and values underlying industrial labour conflict in Temirtau. But even when traditionalization is effectively validated by reference to shared values and traditions, its efficacy in labour conflict is no forgone conclusion. Actors realize that their contemporary concerns and struggles can only partially be captured by the realm of tradition when they are, in effect, about labour and power.

Notes

1. All quotes are translated from the Russian by the author. Except where noted, all words in italics are in Russian.
2. Mr Kamzabaev wished his real name to be given in this article. All other names of informants are given as initials.
3. Cf. Brumann's (2011) review of anthropological debates on tradition.
4. Due to its massive size and output (the largest steel mill in Central Asia, with 40,000 employees, and 6 million tons of annual steel production in its Soviet heyday), Karmet alone accounted for a large part of Kazakhstan's gross domestic product (Karaganda 1986) and was the most important outlet for raw materials produced in the coal and iron mining region of Karaganda.
5. That is, those related and those unrelated to the factory were divided over their jobs and over the evaluation of the environmental costs to society attached to these jobs (Prilutskaya 2016).
6. For similar trends in Russia, see Ashwin and Clarke (2003).
7. In the world of Soviet industry, veterans enjoyed public recognition and privileges, especially if they had been better-qualified elite workers, and even more so if they had come from families with labour dynasties. The status of a labour veteran could be achieved by any worker after many years working in the steel plant, and it was usually reached near retirement. Labour dynasties were those with members of several generations who worked or had worked in the plant (Lane 1981, 115; Ashwin 1999; Kesküla 2018).
8. Shop floor management turnover had dramatically increased. In the Soviet era, plant managers kept their positions for long periods, ideally transmitting them along the lines of labour dynasties.
9. In August 2018 a corporate Kurban-ait was held at the city mosque under the aegis of a newly established Department for Ethnocultural Affairs at ArcelorMittal Temirtau. Reporting in the company journal makes no mention of any speeches touching on labour issues. Photographs of the event show mostly Kazakhs in a sober, religious meeting, without the presence of either Soviet veterans or management (Tikhonov 2018).

Acknowledgements

Early versions of this manuscript were presented at the ESCAS 2015 conference in Zürich and at the 'Practices of Traditionalization in Central Asia' workshop at Konstanz University in November 2017. I thank the editors of this special issue, the journal editor and the three anonymous reviewers for their valuable comments on the manuscript. Fieldwork (September 2013 to May 2014 and August to September 2014) benefited immensely from the research assistance of Xeniya Prilutskaya.

Disclosure statement

No potential conflict of interest was reported by the author.

Funding

Research was funded by the Max Planck Institute for Social Anthropology.

ORCID

Tommaso Trevisani http://orcid.org/0000-0001-9092-030X

References

Adams, L. 2010. *The Spectacular State: Culture and National Identity in Uzbekistan*. Durham and London: Duke University Press.

Ashwin, S. 1999. *Russian Workers: The Anatomy of Patience*. Manchester: Manchester University Press.

Ashwin, S., and S. Clarke. 2003. *Russian Trade Unions and Industrial Transition*. London: Palgrave.

Bacon, E. 1966. *Central Asians under Russian Rule: A Study in Culture Change*. Ithaca and London: Cornell University Press.

Barnes, S. 2011. *Death and Redemption: The Gulag and the Shaping of Soviet Society*. New Jersey: Princeton University Press.

Burawoy, M. 2002. "Transition without Transformation: Russia's Involutionary Road to Capitalism." In *Locating Capitalism in Time and Space: Global Restructurings, Politics, and Identity*, edited by D. Nugent, 290–310. Stanford, CA: Stanford University Press.

Beyer, J. 2006. "Revitalisation, Invention and Continued Existence of the Kyrgyz Aksakal Courts: Listening to Pluralistic Accounts of History." *Journal of Legal Pluralism and Unofficial Law* 38: 141–176. doi:10.1080/07329113.2006.10756601

Beyer, J. 2016. *The Force of Custom. Law and the Ordering of Everyday Life in Kyrgyzstan*. Pittsburgh, PA: University of Pittsburgh Press.

Bruman, C. 2011. "Tradition." In *Lexikon der Globalisierung*, edited by F. Kreff, E.-M. Knoll, and A. Gingrich, 381–383. Bielefeld: transcript.

Buttino, M. 2015. *Samarcanda: Storia di una città dal 1945 a oggi*. Roma: Viella.

Collier, S. 2011. *Post-Soviet Social. Neoliberalism, Social Modernity, Biopolitics*. Princeton and Oxford: Princeton University Press.

Csikszentmihalyi, M. 1990. *Flow: The Psychology of Optimal Experience*. New York: Harper and Row.

Dubuisson, E.-M. 2014. "Dialogic Authority: Kazakh Aitys Poets and Their Patrons." In *Ethnographies of the State in Central Asia. Performing Politics*, edited by M. Reeves, J. Rasanayagam, and J. Beyer, 55–77. Bloomington, IN: Indiana University Press.

Dulatbekov, N. O. 2012. *Karlag*. Karaganda: "Bolashak" Karaganda University.

Edele, M. 2008. *Soviet Veterans of World War II: A Popular Movement in an Authoritarian Society. 1941–1991*. Oxford: Oxford University Press.

Grant, B. 1996. *In the Soviet House of Culture: A Century of Perestroikas*. Princeton, NJ: Princeton University Press.

Guyer, J. 2007. "Prophecy and the Near Future: Thoughts on Macroeconomic, Evangelical, and Punctuated Time." *American Ethnologist* 34 (3): 409–421. doi:10.1525/ae.2007.34.3.409

Hann, C., and J. Parry. 2018. *Industrial Labor on the Margins of Capitalism: Precarity, Class and the Neoliberal Subject*. New York and Oxford: Berghahn.

Herzfeld, M. 1997. *Cultural Intimacy. Social Poetics in the Nation-State*. New York: Routledge.
Hobsbawm, E. J., and T. Ranger, eds. 1983. *The Invention of Tradition*. Cambridge: Cambridge University Press.
Igmen, A. 2012. *Speaking Soviet with an Accent: Culture and Power in Kyrgyzstan*. Pittsburgh: University of Pittsburgh Press.
Karaganda. 1986. *Karagandiskaya Oblast' Enciklopediya*. Alma-Ata: Kazakhskoy Sovetskoy Enciklopedii.
Kesküla, E. 2018. "Miners and Their Children: The Remaking of the Soviet Working Class in Kazakhstan." In *Industrial Labor on the Margins of Capitalism: Precarity, Class and the Neoliberal Subject*, edited by C. Hann, and J. Parry, 61–84. New York and Oxford: Berghahn.
Krader, L. 1963. *Peoples of Central Asia*. Bloomington: Indiana University.
Laruelle, M. 2007. *"Wiedergeburt per Dekret. Nationsbildung in Zentralasien." Osteuropa* 57 (8–9): 139–154.
Lane, C. 1981. *The Rites of Rulers: Ritual in Industrial Society – The Case of Russia*. Cambridge: Cambridge University Press.
Levin, T. 1999. *The Hundred Thousand Fools of God. Musical Travels in Central Asia (and Queens, New York)*. Bloomington: Indiana University Press.
Liu, M. 2012. *Under Solomon's Throne: Uzbeks Visions of Renewal in Osh*. Pittsburgh, PA: University of Pittsburgh Press.
Martin, V. 2001. *Law and Custom in the Steppe: The Kazakhs of the Middle Horde and Russian Colonialism in the Nineteenth Century*. Richmond: Curzon.
Massicard, E., and T. Trevisani. 2003. "The Uzbek Mahalla: Between State and Society." In *Central Asia: Aspects of Tradition*, edited by T. Everett-Heath, 205–218. New York: Routledge/Curzon.
Moscaritolo, A. 2012. "Almaty as a New Kazakh City: Kazakhisation of Urban Spaces After Independence." In *Changing Urban Landscapes: Eastern Europe and Post-Soviet Cities Since 1989*, edited by M. Buttino, 23–58. Roma: Viella.
Mrozowicki, A. 2011. *Coping with Social Change: Life Strategies of Workers in Poland's New Capitalism*. Leuven: University Press.
Muehlebach, A. 2017. "The Body of Solidarity: Heritage, Memory, and Materiality in Post-Industrial Italy." *Comparative Studies in Society and History* 59 (1): 96–126. doi:10.1017/S0010417516000542
Mühlfried, F. 2006. *Postsowjetische Feiern. Das Georgische Bankett im Wandel*. Stuttgart: ibidem-Verlag.
Munck, R. 2013. "The Precariat: A View from the South." *Third World Quarterly* 34 (5): 747–762. doi:10.1080/01436597.2013.800751
Neilson, B., and N. Rossiter. 2008. "Precarity as a Political Concept, or, Fordism as Exception." *Theory, Culture and Society* 25 (7–8): 51–72. doi:10.1177/0263276408097796
Poliakov, S. 1992. *Everyday Islam: Religion and Tradition in Rural Central Asia*. London: M.E. Sharpe.
Prilutskaya, X. 2016. Juggling Risk: Lay Perceptions of Ecological and Health Risk in Post-Soviet Mono-industrial Temirtau. Master thesis. Nazarbayev University, Astana. http://nur.nu.edu.kz/handle/123456789/1674.
Rajković, I. 2017. "For an Anthropology of the Demoralized: State pay, Mock-Labour, and Unfreedom in a Serbian Firm." *Journal of the Royal Anthropological Institute* 24: 47–70. doi:10.1111/1467-9655.12751
Rasanayagam, J. 2011. *Islam in Post-Soviet Uzbekistan. The Morality of Experience*. Cambridge: Cambridge University Press.
Reeves, M., J. Rasanayagam, and J. Beyer. 2014. *Ethnographies of the State in Central Asia. Performing Politics*. Bloomington, IN: Indiana University Press.
Ringel, F. 2018. *Back to the Postindustrial Future: An Ethnography of Germany's Fastest-Shrinking City*. Oxford & New York: Berghahn Books.
Rogers, D. 2006. "How to Be a Khoziain in a Transforming State: State Formation and the Ethics of Governance in Post-Soviet Russia." *Comparative Studies in Society and History* 48 (4): 915–945. doi:10.1017/S001041750600034X
Roy, O. 1997. *La nouvelle Asie centrale ou la fabrication des nations*. Paris: Seuil.
Sahlins, M. 1999. "Two or Three Things That I Know about Culture." *Journal of the Royal Anthropological Institute* 5 (3): 399–421. doi:10.2307/2661275

Sanchez, A. 2012. "Deadwood and Paternalism: Rationalizing Casual Labour in an Indian Company Town." *Journal of the Royal Anthropological Institute* 18: 808–827. doi:10.1111/j.1467-9655.2012.01793.x

Scott, J. 1985. *Weapons of the Weak: Everyday Forms of Peasant Resistance*. New Haven, CT: Yale University Press.

Tikhonov, A. 2018. "Za obshim dastarkhanom." *Temirtauskiy Metallurg* 36:6.

Trevisani, T. 2015. "Transformatsiia industrial'nogo rabochego klassa: metallurgi goroda Temirtau." In *Materials of International Scientific-Practical Conference Devoted to the 90th Anniversary of E.A. Buketov*, 590–595. Karaganda: Karaganda State University.

Trevisani, T. 2016. "Under Suspicious Eyes: Work and Fieldwork in a Steel Plant in Kazakhstan." *Zeitschrift für Ethnologie* 141 (2): 281–297.

Trevisani, T. 2018. "Work, Precarity and Resistance: Company and Contract Labor in Kazakhstan's Former Soviet Steel Town." In *Industrial Labor on the Margins of Capitalism: Precarity, Class and the Neoliberal Subject*, edited by C. Hann, and J. Parry, 85–110. New York and Oxford: Berghahn.

Trevisani, T., and E. Kesküla. 2016. *Longing for the "ideal"* khozyain *(owner): Visions of good management and leadership in a steel and coal company in Kazakhstan*. Paper presented at the EASA 2016 conference, Milano Bicocca, 20–23 July 2016.

Willis, P. 1977. *Learning to Labor: How Working-Class Kids get Working-Class Jobs*. Saxon House, UK: Columbia University Press.

Yurchak, A. 2006. *Everything was Forever, Until it Was No More. The Last Soviet Generation*. Princeton, NJ: Princeton University Press.

Appropriating and contesting 'traditional Islam': Central Asian students at the Russian Islamic University in Tatarstan

Dominik Müller

ABSTRACT
Based on an ethnographic case study of an Islamic university in Russia, I examine how the state-implemented and bureaucratized traditionalization of Islam in Russia affects the everyday life of Central Asian students and how this project 'from above' is entangled with their coping strategies. I show how religious education has become a resource for the state as well as for young students and their parents. The Russian state uses these official religious institutions to control the Muslim population by creating and promoting a state-approved version of 'traditional Islam' and producing official religious specialists. For the young Muslim students, however, Islamic education provides, in addition to religious knowledge, access to networks, social security and new economic opportunities. It thereby offers a way to cope with the uncertainty caused by high unemployment rates and other socio-economic difficulties among young people.

Introduction

Russia's largest mosque, after more than a decade under construction, was ceremonially inaugurated by Russian president Vladimir Putin – flanked by Recep Tayyip Erdogan and Mahmoud Abbas and a number of other honorary guests – on 23 September 2015 in Moscow. The Moscow Cathedral Mosque (*Moskovskaia sobornaia mechet*) accommodates approximately 10,000 people on three floors and replaces the much smaller two-storey mosque which was built in 1904. In his inauguration speech, Putin emphasized the status of Islam as 'one of Russia's traditional religions', stressing the role 'traditional' Islamic institutions play in the fight against extremism. At first sight, the president's words sound like the typical rhetoric of a statesman who calls people to interreligious peace and national unity on a prestigious, official occasion. However, with a closer look at the content of the speech and the mosque opening, one can recognize that the event reflects the state's current policy approach to Islam more generally.

Terms like 'traditional Islam' (*traditsionnyi islam*) are much more than mere phrases of empathy; they are also very concrete and powerful discursive tools of governance. Since the second half of the 2000s, the Russian government has started emphasizing Islam as one of Russia's 'traditional religions', facilitating what I will analyse in this article as a 'traditionalization project from above'. However, this traditionalization project, which exhibits a path dependency on similar projects undertaken in the Russian imperial and Soviet eras, is not restricted to the discursive level of government rhetoric but also manifests itself in distinct institutions, such as laws, educational institutions and bodies of religious administration. It thereby has concrete consequences for the everyday religious practices of Muslims in Russia.

Despite the clear importance of this phenomenon, however, there are few studies that deal with the immediate consequences of the traditionalization project for the quotidian lives of Muslims. How do ordinary Muslims perceive and deal with these changes, and what opportunities and challenges do they encounter? What kinds of institutions are being established due to this process of traditionalization, and how are people navigating within these official organizations? These questions are especially interesting for scholars of Central Asia because a significant proportion of Muslims in Russia are labour migrants from Central Asia. Thus, the question arises as to how this top-down process of traditionalization and the current transformation of the Islamic landscape in Russia influence the migration experiences and religious lives of Central Asian migrants.

This article is based on six months of ethnographic fieldwork conducted from 2012 to 2014 in Kazan, the capital of the multi-ethnic and multi-religious Republic of Tatarstan. The fieldwork included participant observation in various Islamic settings, 30 semi-structured interviews, and 15 biographical interviews. The article addresses the questions posed above through case studies of Central Asian students at the Russian Islamic University (RIU) in Kazan, an institution that plays an important role in the official traditionalization project by (re)producing the state-approved version of 'traditional Islam'. By analysing these young Central Asian Muslims' strategies for legitimizing their pursuit of an Islamic education, I show how they react to and appropriate the current transformation of the religious field and how this official institution is intertwined with their migration experiences, coping strategies and imaginaries of the future. As Beyer and Finke (2019, 312, this issue) point out, 'The elites' projects of traditionalization and those of ordinary actors speak to and rely on each other in a rather dialectical way.' I therefore scrutinize the entanglements between the state's project of traditionalization and the 'projects' of my Central Asian interlocutors to analyse what their own understandings and meanings of 'tradition' are and where narratives of tradition come to matter in their everyday lives. This article aims to add a new perspective to the intertwining of religion and tradition, as well as to studies of Central Asian migration to the Russian Federation, especially in relation to religious practices and educational strategies.

Islam, tradition, bureaucracy and the everyday: some theoretical considerations

The term 'traditionalization' points to the fact that 'tradition' is not something essential that exists in the world as such, but something that is produced consciously or unconsciously, a social, political or discursive practice that defines and renders such things as norms, values, belief systems and material culture as 'traditional'. For this reason, I use the term to refer to the entirety of policy measures and practices of governmentality by the Russian state that aim to render Islam 'traditional'.[1]

As a state practice, the traditionalization project is implemented through the institutionalization and bureaucratization of Islam, processes that have a long history in Russia, as I shall demonstrate. In contrast to the Russian Orthodox Church, in which authority is highly structured and hierarchical, authority relations in Islam are somewhat ambiguous and complex, since from a theological perspective Islam 'lacks' the centralized leadership and authority usually associated with Christianity. However, as Müller and Steiner (2018, 4) point out, in most Muslim countries – and also to a certain extent in countries with a relevant Muslim minority – 'hierarchical bodies that make authoritative decisions regarding Islam and its "proper" interpretation and praxis exist'. These religious bureaucracies administer and govern the religious affairs within the state through a variety of interlinked organizations and personnel, (ideally) differentiated according to their field of expertise. To govern belief and practice, the bureaucratization of Islam operates through standardization and formalization, leading to a specific bureaucratic language that translates belief and practice into codes, symbols and procedures and establishes a classificatory power for the relevant state actor (Müller 2017; Müller and Steiner 2018). Thus, the bureaucratization of Islam 'represents a technique of power … [that] aims to erase ambiguities, grey zones, and unregulated spheres' (Müller and Steiner 2018, 14) by imposing 'simple categorical schemes' (Graeber 2012) or 'state simplifications' (Scott 1996) on the society. As I will show in this article, the term 'traditional Islam' in Putin's speech represents one of these 'state simplifications' and has become an important part of the bureaucratic language in the Russian Federation.

According to Müller and Steiner (2018) these 'standardised categorical schemes diffuse into society and become appropriated by social actors and institutions' (14) and 'are increasingly interiorized as natural and, therefore, as authentic among Muslim communities' (5). Hence it is important to focus on the everyday to understand the social life of these bureaucratic categories in the Muslim community. This focus is also crucial to comprehend how religious belief and practice are entangled with other dimensions of an individual's life. In a critical review of the anthropology of Islam, Schielke (2010) noted that 'there is too much Islam in the anthropology of Islam' (2). He criticized ethnographies of the lives of Muslims for often privileging devout persons in pious settings, because doing so risks reproducing 'Islam as the supreme guideline of all fields of life' (2). He concluded that if 'we want to understand what it means to live a Muslim life, then we need a grounded and nuanced understanding of what it means to live a life', and argued for 'an existential and ethnographic approach that accounts for the motivations, experiences, complexities and ambiguities of everyday lives'. As I will show in this article, these ambiguities derive from competing imaginaries and perceptions of what one's life should look like – Schielke calls these competing ideas 'grand schemes' – and the different ways one navigates the complexity of the everyday. Taking these ambiguities as a starting point to analyse the life stories of my interlocutors, in the following section I examine how the category of 'traditional Islam' has found its way into state institutions. I then analyse, on the basis of three case studies, whether and how this category diffuses into the quotidian lives of Central Asian students and how the concept of 'traditional Islam' is negotiated.

From 'tolerated' to 'traditional' religion – a genealogy of Islamic bureaucracy

The first centuries after Ivan Grozny conquered the Tatar Khanate in 1552, which represent the beginning of Russian Orthodox rule over the empire's Muslim subjects, were driven by a minority policy of national integration. This meant (forced) conversion to Christianity, cultural assimilation of the subordinated Muslim population, and the drastic reduction of the Islamic infrastructure (Faller 2011; Rorlich 1986; Yemelianova 1999, 2003).

The situation of the Muslim population improved with the rule of Tsarina Catherine the Great, who in 1773 issued the Tolerance Edict, which was intended to assure toleration of the religious beliefs and practices of all major religious groups in the empire (Graney 2010; Kappeler and Clayton 2013). This new policy, which sought to transform religious authority in the various religious communities into an instrument of imperial rule, also marks the beginning of the bureaucratization of Islam. In 1788 the first Islamic administrative body, the Orenburg Mohameddan Spiritual Assembly (*Orenburgskoie magometanskoie dukhovnoie sobraniie*), was established in Orenburg. This new Islamic administration, led by a government-approved *mufti*, and the related policies had serious impacts on the Muslim communities by creating new rules for the construction of mosques and introducing bureaucratic procedures for the appointment of religious scholars (*ulema*) and prayer leaders (*imams*) (Garipova 2013). Furthermore, the very function of these authorities within the Muslim community was altered by assigning new tasks with a mainly bureaucratic character to them, such as the registration of marriages and the administration of civil registers. This shift of tasks to the social-administrative field converted religious scholars into 'state bureaucrats' (Garipova 2013, 36). This had the effect of transforming Islam from a 'hostile' religion and ideology of resistance into a 'tolerated' and controlled religion through state techniques of bureaucratization. Furthermore, as an important part of imperial governmentality, this shift became an effective way to govern religious minorities by co-opting religious leaders who were loyal to the state.

The status of Islam changed once more with the establishment of the Soviet Union, where religion was seen as an ideological opponent of communist ideas and the Soviet state. The Islamic infrastructure was drastically reduced to two teaching institutes in Uzbekistan and not more than 400 official mosques throughout the whole USSR, strictly controlled by four Muslim Spiritual Administrations, in Ufa, Baku, Makhachkala and Tashkent (Kemper and Bustanov 2012). However, the category of 'religion' remained an important part of governmentality because 'religion', along with language, was the main attribute used to classify the population into different ethno-religious nations (Kappeler and Clayton 2013). So even though the Soviet regime aimed to eradicate religion, anti-religion policies had 'unintentionally created nations and a sense of ethno-national identity that was inextricably bound up with religious belonging' (McBrien 2017, 25).

Under the politics of Gorbachev in the 1980s, the restrictions on private and public religious life were abolished. As a consequence, churches and mosques were built and religious organizations formed across the country (Mukhametshin 2010). Religion became even more relevant after the collapse of the Soviet Union, as it played an important role in the nation-building processes of the newly independent states on the territory of the former Soviet Union (Makarov and Mukhametshin 2003). Once again religion as a sense of belonging, rather than an internal belief system, became an important category for both political mobilization and the governance and control of the Muslim population, as is detailed in the next section.

Defining and teaching 'traditional Islam'

At the beginning of the 1990s only a few institutions for Islamic practice and teaching remained in the Russian Federation (Malashenko and Nuritova 2009). To counter this dearth, a system of Islamic education in the Volga–Ural region was created with substantial financial aid and personnel from various Saudi Arabian, Turkish, Egyptian and other foreign Islamic funds, organizations and movements (Mukhametshin 2010, 57). The combination of foreign support and initiatives from local actors led to the establishment of numerous mosques and educational institutions, as well as to a highly heterogeneous Islamic organizational landscape in which a large number of organizations, movements and actors competed for followers in the marketplace of ideas (Garaev 2017, 199). The foreign sponsors had full control over the Islamic educational system until the mid-1990s, when Russian authorities stopped their activities by prohibiting foreign financial involvement. The Russian state was then forced to build up its own system of religious education and to compensate for the sudden loss of foreign investment by creating state programmes to support 'the traditionalist version of Islam at home' (Garaev 2017, 198). This brings us back to the meaning of 'traditional Islam' from the perspective of the elites.

At the beginning of the speech mentioned in the introduction, Putin emphasized the status of Islam as 'one of Russia's traditional religions ... under our country's law' (Kremlin.ru 2017). In the course of his speech, Putin further elaborated on what he understands by 'traditional Islam', the values it embodies and the institutions that represent it. He stressed the humanistic values of 'traditional Islam', such as compassion, justice and care for others. At the same time, however, he asserted a clear distinction between 'traditional Islam', geographically bounded within the Russian Federation, and those Islamic movements and ideas that come from abroad, blaming them for domestic problems. Once again – as we have seen in the approach to religion in the tsarist era as well as in the Soviet period – religion in the guise of 'traditional Islam' is constructed as a sense of belonging and loyalty *vis-à-vis* the state. The 'traditionalization of Islam' in the Russian Federation is, therefore, not so much a theological endeavour as it is a political project, in which the loyalty of Russia's Muslims to the state is more important than the actual religious teachings. The Russian government thus creates a strong dichotomy between 'traditional Islam', which is considered the good version of Islam, and all other forms, which are seen as potentially dangerous. The idea of a dichotomy between 'good' and 'bad' Islam and between 'good' and 'bad' Muslims (Mamdani 2004) not only relates to the perceived current threats of Islamist organizations such as ISIS, but also reflects the experiences of the 1990s described above, when the Islamic organizational landscape in Russia was dominated by foreign actors. To achieve and uphold this 'dualistic categorization' (Dannreuther 2010), the government expanded the existing Islamic bureaucracy and increased the number of Muslim Spiritual Administrations to 57 in Russia (Kemper and Bustanov 2012). President Putin mentioned another important element of Islamic bureaucracy in his speech: the network of Islamic theological schools, which define, maintain and spread the state-approved 'traditional Islam' through their religious education. This brings us back to the main institution of my case study, the RIU.

The university was founded in 1998 through the cooperation of the Spiritual Administration of Muslims of the Republic of Tatarstan, the Russian Council of Muftis, and the Institute of History of the Academy of Sciences of Tatarstan, and was officially registered as a non-state institution of higher professional education. Over the years, the number of students at the RIU has increased steadily: from 24 in 1998 to more than 1,000 in 2018.

Approximately 60% of the students are local, 20% from other parts of the Russian Federation, and another 20% from foreign countries, half of these coming from Central Asia.

In 2007 RIU became the first Islamic educational institution in Russia to receive state accreditation from the Ministry of Education and Science. At that time, the university was divided into two teaching facilities operating in parallel: the Russian Islamic Institute and Kazan Islamic University.[2] The Russian Islamic Institute offers educational programmes based on state educational standards, granting state-recognized (secular) bachelor's and master's degrees in theology, with specializations in Islamic theology, Islamic economy, Islamic journalism and linguistics. In contrast, Kazan Islamic University offers programmes in higher religious education with specializations in Islamic sciences and Qur'anic sciences for personnel of religious organizations. After four years of study at Kazan Islamic University, graduates can obtain the degree of *imam khatib*, which authorizes them to work in a mosque as an imam. Due to this dual structure the university educates not only religious specialists but also professionals at the intersection of the secular and religious spheres. This is one example of how the Islamic bureaucracy reproduces itself by training specialized personnel in a variety of fields, who are afterwards able to expand the reach of the traditionalization project. This also shows that the traditionalization transcends religion and entangles it with the social and economic fields.

This dual structure also makes the institution very attractive for potential and current students, as it allows them to pursue an Islam-related subject in their studies and still obtain a state-recognized diploma. In addition, the more applied subjects, such as Islamic economics and journalism, are very popular among my interlocutors because they qualify them to work in emerging fields of the job market. I now turn to the analysis of my interlocutors' life stories to make visible how the elites' traditionalization project is entangled with the projects of my interlocutors.

Alisher and the entanglements of the religious and the secular

The story of Alisher (20 years old), who was born in rural Tajikistan and is now in his fourth year at RIU studying Islamic sciences, begins with the migration experience of his mother. Farkhonda, who divorced her husband when Alisher was still very young, has lived in Kazan for more than 10 years. She went with her daughter Gulrukhsor to Kazan as a labour migrant, following her older son Firuz, who had already been working there for several years. Upon her arrival, a friend who had a small shop in a local bazaar on the outskirts of Kazan hired her. After working there for several years, she was able to save some money and, together with her older son, open her own market stall for clothes in another bazaar in Kazan. All this time Alisher lived with his father in Tajikistan, because he had to finish school first, and his mother was not sure how successful their small business in Kazan would be. It was easier for her to deal with the uncertainty without her youngest son staying with her. After Alisher finished school in 2010, his mother decided that he should join the rest of the family in Kazan. She had been looking at a number of institutions of higher education in Kazan for him and finally decided in favour of RIU.

The first thing that intrigued me about Alisher's life story, which he told me when I met him at RIU in 2013, was that his mother had made the decision regarding his educational future. As I later found out, Alisher's case was in fact quite common. In all but one case, the parents of my Central Asian interlocutors played a significant role in the decision-making processes related to their studies at RIU. Like Alisher's mother, other parents strongly encouraged their children to study at a religious institution. This raises the question of why parents are so fond of the idea of having their children get an Islamic education. When I asked Alisher about this, his first explanation was 'tradition':

> This is very usual in Tajikistan.... It's our tradition.... Most of the time, the parents [don't] just send one kid to get an Islamic education, but at least two or three.... And sometimes all of the children get some kind of Islamic education.

In this quote, 'tradition' is used as justification for his mother's decision as well as an explanation for his own overt religious practice. This use of 'tradition' is widespread and was usually the first explanation given when I asked my interlocutors about their motivations for engaging in the Islamic field. This common usage can be linked to two motives: on the one hand, it is recourse to the (imagined and also promoted) religious history and 'tradition' in Central Asia (Epkenhans 2010), as well as to the growing popularity of religious education in Tajikistan (Stephan 2010). On the other hand, it is a way of distancing one's religious practice from other forms of religious practice or orientation that are considered 'non-traditional' and potentially dangerous.[3] My interlocutors thus upheld the very dichotomy of traditional versus non-traditional Islam that is promoted and reproduced through the Islamic bureaucracy in Russia. On numerous occasions in our conversations, Alisher emphasized that it is not always easy to live in Russia as a Central Asian. In everyday life, one encounters prejudices, racism and discrimination against migrant workers, and the fact that he is religious and studies at an Islamic university compounds these difficulties. He deals with the mistrust and suspicion by explaining and emphasizing that he is studying at an 'official religious institution' and is 'practising a traditional form of Islam'. According to Rasanayagam (2014, 3), categories and classifications produced within 'state political imaginaries' – such as 'traditional Islam' – create possibilities for religious expression. By stressing the 'traditional' dimension when he talks about his studies or his religious practice, Alisher puts a stamp of approval on his activities. This practice of referring to official Islamic institutions or 'traditional' and state-approved forms of religious practice to emphasize the legitimacy of one's own religiosity can also be found in other countries, such as Turkey, Egypt and Indonesia, where religious affairs are controlled and administered by a strong central authority with an Islamic bureaucracy (Hart 2013; Müller 2017). The example illustrates how these constructed categories permeate everyday life and how they become appropriated by Muslims themselves. However, this does not necessarily mean that the categories are also internalized as natural and authentic among the Muslim community, as Müller and Steiner (2018) have argued. In the case of Alisher, it was much more a (rhetorical) strategy for coping with his position as a Muslim migrant in Russia, an identity that is often doubly stigmatized.

However, the question as to why Alisher's mother decided to send him to an Islamic university has not yet been fully answered. When I asked Alisher about this, he said:

> My mother wanted someone in our family to have a religious education.... A religious education is a good thing ... because if something happens, the person with a religious education will be able to judge the situation and solve the problem. Islamic education is not just about knowledge; it's also about upbringing [*vospitaniie*]!

But to fully describe the reasons and motivations behind his mother's decision, I have to introduce more of Alisher's family history. Like Alisher's mother, many Central Asian parents emphasized that they do not have as much time as they may wish to raise their children, especially as many family members live apart because of labour migration. Alisher's mother works from early morning until late evening, and Alisher's father still lives in Tajikistan, so the children are on their own most of the time. This situation leads many parents to fear that their children will not get the proper upbringing (*vospitaniie*) necessary to become a good person. As Alisher's mother once said, 'While Russia is a good place to earn money and do business, it's not such a good place to raise your children properly.' Furthermore, they do not trust public schools to provide a proper upbringing, which is a result of the transformation of the educational system in post-Soviet Russia and the still widespread romanticization of the Soviet past, when the socialist state purportedly did provide a proper upbringing through its various institutions (Imbrogno 1986). This distrust of the educational system is not a peculiarity of Central Asian migrants in Russia; it can also often be found in their countries of origin. In her analysis of the growing popularity of private religious lessons in Dushanbe, Stephan (2010, 475) has illustrated how Islamic education serves 'as a powerful tool to socialize urban Muslim youth into the existing social order'. Furthermore, the fear that the public school system in Russia cannot provide a proper upbringing and education is not limited to Central Asian parents; it is widespread in Russian society (Suleymanova 2015).

In many parents' opinions, the burden of providing a proper upbringing today therefore lies foremost with the family. As we have seen in the case of Alisher, parents hope that an Islamic education will teach morality, modesty, good manners and the skills needed to cope with the problems of everyday life. As such, Islamic education becomes a coping strategy to deal with the migration experience. For many parents it also represents an alternative mode of upbringing, offering normative and moral guidelines for their children.

Now I shift the focus to Alisher's perspective and how his mother's decision to have him attend RIU placed him right in the middle of the traditionalization project, which has resulted in both opportunities and limitations.

Alisher shares a dormitory room on campus with three other RIU students, but he tries to visit his family in Kazan twice a week. Usually, the whole family gathers at his mother's place to eat *plov*, a Central Asian rice dish. His older brother, who no longer lives with his mother, brings along his wife and sometimes other friends of the family. During dinner, Alisher tells his family what he has learned at university, and after dinner he regularly gives religious lectures, tries to answer the family's questions regarding religious practice or explain different interpretations of Qur'anic verses, and offers advice in everyday matters. As we can see in these weekly family gatherings, religious education can also have an influence on the expanded family of the students. Through his studies, Alisher has acquired moral and religious authority in his family, though he is its youngest member. He is able to transform his studies at RIU into social capital, elevating his position in the family hierarchy and his close environment. Again, this dynamic is quite common among Central Asian students at the university. Many students start sharing their religious knowledge with their families immediately after beginning their studies by reading and interpreting the Qur'an for their families and their peer group. Through their Islamic education, they not only raise their position in the hierarchy of the family but also improve their social mobility in the wider societal context. This religious and social capital can even transcend the religious sphere. As Stephan (2010, 473) has shown, religiosity and religious education can make young Muslims more attractive marriage partners, because 'decency and morality (*odob*) in combination with a good education are considered as a guarantee for successful marriage arrangements'.

This practice of teaching and sharing knowledge with their families, relatives and peer group can also lead to conflicts, as Alisher often mentioned during our conversations:

> Sometimes people around me don't like it when I teach them. They have their own interpretations and ideas, which are often based on their tradition and are not always really Islamic. They often refer to themselves as traditional Muslims, but they do not practise at all. They are just ethnic Muslims.

This differentiation between 'ethnic Muslims' and 'practising Muslims' was a very common strategy of my Central Asian interlocutors to distinguish themselves from other Muslims who, according to them, have not received a 'proper religious education' or 'did not understand or practise Islam the right way'. In this line of argumentation, the expressions 'ethnic Muslim' and 'traditional Muslim' were often used interchangeably, imbuing 'tradition' with a derogatory connotation. While at the beginning of my research Alisher, and many of my other interlocutors, used the category 'traditional Muslim' as a self-description to legitimize their religious practice, over time a substantial critique of the very concept of being a 'traditional Muslim' emerged in his narrative. His critique, and that of many of his fellow students, revolved around the question of what it actually means to be a Muslim. For most of my interlocutors, being a Muslim is defined by religious practice and belief, and they accuse the 'traditional Muslims' of reducing their faith to a sense of belonging. These competing understandings of being a Muslim reflect the state approaches to religion described earlier. Both the Russian Empire and the Soviet Union institutionally cultivated this reduction of religion to a sense of belonging as an instrument of governmentality. Since most of my interlocutors' parents were socialized in the Soviet period, they internalized this Soviet way of being Muslim, which can lead to serious intergenerational conflicts within the family.[4]

Although Alisher is studying Islamic sciences and will therefore be entitled to work as an imam after graduation, he is not planning to become a religious specialist. As he mentioned several times, he is studying first and foremost for his private life, not for his professional future. According to Alisher, it would also be very difficult for him, as a Tajik, to work as an imam in a mosque in Tatarstan, since most of the imams are Tatars, and the mosque community would probably not accept him as an imam. Furthermore, in August 2016, the Spiritual Administration of Muslims of Tatarstan decided that Tatar is the only language allowed for Friday sermons (*khutba*) in mosques throughout the Republic of Tatarstan. This change in legislation is another obstacle to non-Tatar-speaking students becoming imams.[5]

Since Alisher does not see his professional future in the religious field, he is also studying part-time at a vocational school for construction-related professions. Several of his fellow students at RIU are also studying there. This strategy of combining a religious and a secular education is actively supported by the university. In fact, RIU has bilateral agreements with several secular educational institutions in and around Kazan. Through these agreements, the students are allowed to study for free at other educational institutions. Alisher's example also shows how religious education at the university can give the students access to networks outside of the religious field, and how the religious and the secular spheres are entangled through the traditionalization project.

Welcome to 'Muslim Disneyland': Ansar and the contestation of 'tradition'

One afternoon I went with Ansar, an Uzbek student from Kyrgyzstan studying in the Theology Department, to the Kul Sharif mosque, in the Kazan Kremlin. As soon as we entered the Kremlin, which is both the main government district and one of the major tourist attractions in Kazan, we realized that the place was quite crowded. I mentioned how much I liked the Kul-Sharif Mosque, with its sky-blue domes and six minarets, because it exudes a special atmosphere. Ansar looked at me a little surprised at first and then said, 'Welcome to Russia's Muslim Disneyland!' I was amused and amazed by this statement and asked him what he meant by it. He explained that the mosque had become a popular tourist destination over the past few years, and added:

> I appreciate that they [the government] are investing money, but I am not sure about their intentions. For whom are they doing this – for us Muslims or for the tourists? During some prayer times, you can find more tourists in the Kul-Sharif Mosque than believers, and when they are watching you during prayers you feel like an animal in a zoo. They always talk about their Islamic tradition, but is it really about the religion or is it just to show off, to attract tourists, to give them a little touch of the 'orient'?

Like many other students, Ansar was quite sceptical about the state's involvement in the religious field through investments in Muslim infrastructure, as well as about the increasing commercialization of the Islamic heritage of the region. According to him, the 'Islamic tradition' and 'traditional Islam' had become brands used to attract tourists from all over Russia and to sell souvenirs. On the other hand, he often criticized the official label 'traditional Islam' for excluding other forms of Islamic practice and belief, usually by stigmatizing them as 'Wahhabi' (see also Abashin 2006). The example of Ansar shows that the traditionalization project is also critically received: even though bureaucratized forms of Islam are often interiorized as 'natural' and 'authentic' (Müller and Steiner 2018, 5), the classificatory power and involvement of the state can also lead to detachment from constructed categories like 'traditional Islam'. In their introduction to this special issue, Beyer and Finke (2019, 317) note that new classifications have to make sense to the actors themselves and that 'the further away from established ideas it is, the more effort has to be spent to implement it'. Puzzled by Ansar's criticism of the official Muslim infrastructure – of which the university where he studies is a central part – I asked him on another occasion how satisfied he was with his studies. After considering my question, he said:

> It's okay. The teachers are friendly; they also have knowledge and try to do their best, teaching us as much as they can. But to be honest, we [Uzbeks] have much better methods of teaching; our teachers teach one-to-one – it's like with a *repetitor* [tutor]. We Uzbeks have a long Islamic history and famous historical centres of religious teaching. On the other hand, [the teaching of] secular knowledge [*svetskiie znaniia*] is much better here at the university.

This comment requires further contextualization. Like Ansar, many of my Central Asian interlocutors had already received some form of Islamic education earlier in their lives. It was therefore quite natural for them to compare the education they had received in

Central Asia with the education they were getting at RIU. In these comparisons, the students, especially those of Uzbek origin, often stated that the Islamic education in their countries of origin was better, because their own 'Islamic tradition' was more 'authentic' and more 'historically rooted' than the one in Tatarstan. In doing so, they invoked the 'invented tradition' of their home countries, which is also an important part of post-Soviet nation-building processes in Central Asia (see Beyer and Finke's introduction to this special issue and Akiner 2003). The 'Islamic tradition' in Tatarstan, on the other hand, was seen as more 'corrupted' due to the long coexistence under Russian rule. This criticism is strongly connected to the bureaucratization of Islam in Russia and the people who work within this apparatus, as Ansar explained:

> You know, in the past these people were passionate advocates of communism and functionaries in the party [*apparatchiki*]. Today they have simply changed clothes and are now servants in the Islamic system. It's sometimes very hard to take them seriously.

These prejudices against the new Muslim clergy who are working hand in hand with the state apparatus are widespread and certainly not limited to the Central Asian students at RUI, but can also be found in the wider Tatar community outside the university. This shows again that a highly centralized and bureaucratized system, despite its (classificatory) power, can also lead to alienation from the organizations that embody this bureaucracy and to an erosion or delegitimization of the authority of the persons involved (Müller 2017; Müller and Steiner 2018). As pointed out by Beyer and Finke (2019, 319, this issue), authority does not simply mean enforcing one's individual will or holding a particular office, but is much more an 'effect of a co-emergent practice of legitimization'.

Despite his strong criticism of the Muslim infrastructure and the traditionalization project itself, Ansar stayed at the university because of the secular knowledge (*svetskiie znaniia*) the university offers. At the time of my fieldwork, Ansar decided to change his degree programme from theology to Islamic journalism because he was planning to work for one of the various Muslim publishing houses or broadcasting channels, which are, according to Ansar, flourishing and in need of qualified workers. Ansar's decision and ambitions are, like those of Alisher, entangled with the traditionalization project: the Islamic bureaucracy in Russia includes not only administrative bodies like the muftiates and teaching institutes, but also broadcasting channels such as Alif TV (https://alif.tv), which are able to reach a wider audience.

The example of Ansar shows how state projects of traditionalization can lead to criticism and rejection. This rejection can be based on competing ideas and meanings of 'tradition' (traditional Islam in Tatarstan versus traditional Islam in Uzbekistan), but is also related to the ways these projects are achieved (for example, through the bureaucratization of Islam). However, despite his criticism, Ansar continues to participate in this traditionalization project by studying at an institute of higher education that is implicated in the project and by trying to realize his professional future in an occupational field that is likewise entangled with the project.

My last case study, that of Ismoil, another Tajik student, will show yet another configuration of how the institutions of 'traditional Islam' can be entangled with the coping strategies of Central Asian migrants in Tatarstan.

'The Islamic economy will be big business': Ismoil and the transnational Islamic field

Ismoil is from Tajikistan and is in the fourth year of a bachelor's degree programme in Islamic economics. Ismoil's father is himself an economist who worked his way up from an accountant position in a small shoe factory in urban Tajikistan to become the owner of the company. With the outbreak of the civil war in Tajikistan, their situation changed: Ismoil's father lost the company, and the family was forced to flee the country and decided to go to Saint Petersburg. However, Ismoil's parents could not find jobs in Russia that were suited to their qualifications and were compelled to work as manual labourers, his father on a construction site and his mother as a cleaner for a large company. In contrast to Alisher, it was Ismoil's own decision, not that of his parents, to study at RIU. Nevertheless, his decision-making process is inevitably linked with the family history.

Ismoil was not sure what to do with his future, and he thought for several months about what and where to study. Some years ago, Ismoil travelled from Saint Petersburg to Kazan to visit a relative. On a walk, he passed by RIU and heard a group of students in the yard speaking Tajik. Curious about who these young men were and what they were doing there, he started a conversation. He got along with them very well, and during the remaining three weeks of his holidays in Kazan, Ismoil spent nearly every evening visiting these Tajik students in the university dormitory. After he returned to Saint Petersburg, he informed his parents that he wanted to study at RIU. During my field research, Ismoil told me several times what a great experience it had been for him to meet those students. From the beginning he 'felt a strong connection to them' and it was 'the close relationship between the students', who addressed each other as 'brother' and 'sister', that made him feel 'welcome and safe' outside his family for the first time since they left Tajikistan.

Ismoil had not been very religious before he decided to study at RIU, so this feeling of being integrated into a new and inclusive group was a very important factor in his decision. Most of the students at the university refer to their friends and the teaching staff as their new 'family', the most important peer group and community in their new country. As Stephan (2010, 471) has shown, religious education in Tajikistan plays 'a significant role in the socializing of urban youth in the Muslim community'. In the context of migration, this integrating function of a religious institution becomes even more important and multivalent, as its significance and function often transcend the religious sphere (Schiffauer 2006). For many Central Asian students, the university represents more than a place of religious education; the new community helps them deal with the migration experience by providing information about legal procedures such as obtaining a residence permit, job opportunities and housing possibilities. In other words, RIU and its community provide social security.

Ismoil was furthermore attracted by the available degree programmes, especially those with secular curricula. He always wanted to follow in his father's footsteps and study economics, but doubted whether it would be possible for him. He applied several times to an economics institute in Saint Petersburg, but each time he was rejected because, as he explained, he had 'neither the connections nor the money' to get accepted to such an institute. When Ismoil heard that it would be possible for him to study Islamic economics at RIU, he was very excited and his decision was finally made. An important factor in his decision was his conviction that the Islamic economy is developing into a promising niche in Russia:

> The Islamic economy in Russia will be big business. Now is a good time to get started, because there are still very few specialists in this field. But in the future, it will be big. Russia also joined the OIC and is expanding its relations with Muslim countries such as Malaysia and Indonesia.

Ismoil's assessment is based on the fact that Russia joined the Organisation of Islamic Cooperation (OIC) in 2005 as an observer and has been intensifying and expanding its political and economic relations with the member countries ever since.

Ismoil is also planning to continue his studies at a university in Turkey or Indonesia after he receives his bachelor's degree. His future plans are linked to the bilateral agreements RIU has established with foreign universities in several Muslim countries. Since 2009, RIU has been a member of the Federation of the Universities of the Islamic World (FUIW), an organization working within the framework of the Islamic Educational, Scientific and Cultural Organization (ISESCO). The membership in FUIW allows graduates of RIU to continue their studies in internationally recognized educational centres in Turkey, Malaysia or Indonesia. According to Ismoil, he has always dreamed of going to study in Turkey or Indonesia, but he never believed it could come true, as the Tajik government imposes many restrictions on religious studies abroad.[6] As became clear to me from my conversations with other Tajik students, Ismoil is not the only one who plans to continue his studies at a foreign university after completing his undergraduate studies.

This illustrates how RIU's agreements provide students with the opportunity to circumvent the strict regulations in their countries of origin by first completing a bachelor's degree in Russia and then moving directly from there to a foreign university. As a result, RIU is turning itself into a hub for transnational educational practices, as described by Stephan (2013). Although Ismoil never mentioned any form of 'traditional Islam' in our conversations, his life trajectory and hopes for the future are inevitably entangled with the traditionalization project. Ismoil's story shows that the traditionalization project is not restricted to defining the approved forms of Islamic belief and practice but also transcends the strictly religious field by using Islamic heritage and 'Islamic tradition' to open up new markets and international cooperation, thereby entering the sphere of global economy and politics. It operates not only through restrictions but also by creating incentives to take part in this project and opening up new possibilities.

Conclusion

By scrutinizing the genealogy of Islamic bureaucracy in Russia and combining an institutional approach with the analysis of my Central Asian interlocutors' life stories, I have revealed how these students deal with the ongoing governmental 'traditionalization project' of Islam and how this project is entangled with those of ordinary actors in everyday life. Through the bureaucratization of religion, the classification of 'traditional Islam' has become a powerful discursive tool for the government that not only defines state-approved versions of religious belief, expression and practice but also manifests itself in specific institutions in ways that have concrete consequences for the everyday religious practices of Muslims in Russia.

At the beginning of my fieldwork, most of my interlocutors reproduced the official narrative on 'traditional Islam' to legitimize their own engagement with the religious field or to distance themselves from other versions of religious practice and expression that are not state approved because of the highly controlled and securitized religious landscape. Over time, however, and especially in everyday situations, a more nuanced picture began to emerge. Even though my interlocutors themselves study at an institution that is implicated in the elites' traditionalization project, many of them were highly critical of a number of aspects of the project, ranging from the commercialization and commodification of religion, to the reduction of faith, to a sense of belonging, to the entanglements of religious personnel with the state apparatus. So why are these students participating in this project despite their fundamental disagreements with it, and what does this say about the entanglements between the elites' project of traditionalization and those of ordinary actors?

The story as I have told it permits several conclusions. One would be that the students participate superficially in the elites' project, but in their innermost beings are following their own 'projects' in search of an 'authentic Islam'. Another conclusion would be that the bureaucratization of Islam is so powerful that the hegemonic formations do not allow any course of action other than to participate. I would say that neither of these construals accurately represents the situation. I draw a different conclusion, using Schielke's approach, as described earlier in the article. Taking the ambiguities of everyday life as a starting point to analyse the life stories presented here, I can paint a more nuanced picture of how the traditionalization project affects and is negotiated in daily life. As I have shown, these ambiguities derive from different motivations, ideas and imaginaries of the future that provide meaning and direction in the lives of my interlocutors, such as becoming and being a good Muslim, making a living, starting a career, studying abroad, being a good son, or meeting parents' expectations. Sometimes these grand schemes (Schielke 2010) or 'cultural models' (Beyer and Finke 2019, this issue) are mutually reinforcing, but more often they compete with one another. In any case, they are always derived from and embedded in the local contexts within which people are acting. Understood in this way, participating in and at the same time criticizing the elite's traditionalization project is not a paradox but a strategy for coping with the challenges, restrictions and prejudices one encounters as a young Muslim migrant in Russia. It is also the result of individual negotiations between a person's hopes and aspirations, on the one hand, and the reality of the limitations on his or her own scope of action, on the other hand.

In the academic literature, the governmentality of Islam in post-Soviet spaces is often analysed and depicted with a focus on control, restrictions and coercion. However, as has been shown in this article, the elites' traditionalization project works not only through modes of control or restriction but also through co-optation, namely, by creating incentives to participate in this project. RIU provides applied forms of education and vocational training (for example, Islamic economics, journalism and philology), as well as secular knowledge and connections to other institutions of higher education in Russia and abroad, creating employment opportunities for students in emerging job markets. This shows that the elites' traditionalization project transcends the alleged borders of the religious sphere. For young Muslim students, Islam and an Islamic education provide – in addition to religious knowledge – access to networks, social security and new economic opportunities. I argue, therefore, that we have to bring the agency of young Muslims back into the scholarly analysis, which all too often depicts them as passive actors, more reactive than active, and following a kind of script, be it Islam, a state policy or family expectations. Conceptualizing 'traditionalization' as a practice, as all of the articles in this special issue do, enables us to take into account the complexity and fuzziness of everyday life and to move beyond alleged dichotomies of 'the secular' versus 'the religious', submission versus resistance, and the elites' project of traditionalization versus the projects of ordinary people. The case studies of my Central Asian interlocutors show that these categories dissolve in everyday life and are reconfigured by the actors involved into ever new assemblages of Islam, tradition and bureaucracy to cope with the migration experience.

Notes

1. This process is similar to what Hobsbawm and Ranger (2010 [1983]) described as the 'invention of tradition'. As Beyer and Finke scrutinize the debate on the 'invention of tradition' in the scope of this special issue, I will not further elaborate on it here.
2. Because the university is still usually referred to as the Russian Islamic University in the scientific literature, I will continue to use this name.
3. Beyer (2016) elaborates on 'the force of custom' in the context of Kyrgyzstan.
4. These different modes or understandings of 'being a Muslim' have been analysed by McBrien (2017).
5. The RIU does offer Tatar language courses.
6. Ismoil referred to the Tajik government's campaign, initiated by Emomali Rahmon in 2011, to bring Tajik students who are studying at Islamic universities abroad back to Tajikistan and to implement other laws restricting religious practices.

Acknowledgements

This article is based on ethnographic research carried out from 2012 to 2014 in Kazan (Tatarstan, Russian Federation) and financed by the University of Zurich, Switzerland. The author thanks Judith Beyer, Peter Finke, Johannes Quack, Emanuel Schaeublin, Mascha Schulz, Clémence Jullien, Sandra Bärnreuther, Anne Breubeck, Brian Donahoe and the anonymous reviewers for their helpful comments, and Rafik Mukhametshin, Ibrahim Shaykhabzalov, Danis Garaev, Guzel Suleymanova-Valeeva and Dilyara Suleymanova for their support during the research.

Disclosure statement

No potential conflict of interest was reported by the author.

References

Abashin, S. 2006. "The Logic of Islamic Practice: A Religious Conflict in Central Asia." *Central Asian Survey* 25 (3): 267–286. doi:10.1080/02634930601022542.

Akiner, S. 2003. "The Politicisation of Islam in Postsoviet Central Asia." *Religion, State and Society* 31 (2): 97–122. doi:10.1080/09637490308282.

Beyer, J. 2016. *The Force of Custom: Law and the Ordering of Everyday Life in Kyrgyzstan*. Pittsburgh, PA: University of Pittsburgh Press.

Beyer, J., and Peter, Finke. 2019. "Practices of traditionalization in Central Asia." *Central Asian Survey* 38 (3): 310–328. doi:10.1080/02634937.2019.1636766.

Dannreuther, R. 2010. "Russian Discourses and Approaches to Islam and Islamism." In *Russia and Islam: State, Society and Radicalism*, edited by R. Dannreuther, 9–25. London: Routledge.

Epkenhans, T. 2010. "Muslims without Learning, Clergy without Faith: Institutions of Islamic Learning in the Republic of Tajikistan." In *Islamic Education in the Soviet Union and Its Successor States*, edited by M. Kemper, R. Motika, and S. Reichmuth, 313–348. London: Routledge.

Faller, H. M. 2011. *Nation, Lanuage, Islam: Tatarstan's Sovereignty Movement*. Budapest: Central European University Press.

Garaev, D. 2017. "Islamic Teaching Institutions in the Russian Federation: The Case of Tatarstan." In *Aufbruch zu neuen Ufern: Aufgaben, Problemlagen und Profile einer Islamischen Religionspädagogik im Europäischen Kontext*, edited by Y. Sarıkaya, and F.-J. Bäumer, 197–206. Münster: Waxmann.

Garipova, R. 2013. "The Transformation of the Ulama and the Shari'a in the Volga-Ural Muslim Community under Russian Imperial Rule." (PhD diss.). Princeton University.

Graeber, D. 2012. "Dead Zones of the Imagination: On Violence, Bureaucracy, and Interpretive Labor. The 2006 Malinowski Memorial Lecture." *HAU: Journal of Ethnographic Theory* 2 (2): 105–128. doi:10.14318/hau2.2.007.

Graney, K. E. 2010. *Of Khans and Kremlins : Tatarstan and the Future of Ethno-Federalism in Russia*. Lanham, MD: Lexington Books.

Hart, K. 2013. *And Then We Work for God: Rural Sunni Islam in Western Turkey*. Stanford, CA: Stanford University Press.

Hobsbawm, E. J., and T. O. Ranger, eds. 2010 [1983]. *The Invention of Tradition*. Cambridge: Cambridge University Press.

Imbrogno, S. 1986. "Family Policy in the Soviet Union." *International Journal of Sociology of the Family* 16 (2): 165–180.

Kappeler, A., and A. Clayton. 2013. *The Russian Empire: A Multiethnic History*. Abingdon, Oxon: Routledge, Taylor & Francis Group.

Kemper, M., and A. Bustanov. 2012. "Introduction: Voices of Islam in Russia." In *Islamic Authority and the Russian Language: Studies on Texts from European Russia, the North Caucasus and West Siberia*, edited by A. Bustanov and M. Kemper, 7–26. Amsterdam: Uitgeverij Pegasus.

Kremlin.ru. 2017. 'Moscow's Cathedral Mosque Has Reopened after Reconstruction.' President of Russia. Accessed 16 October 2017. http://en.kremlin.ru/events/president/news/50351.

Makarov, D., and R. Mukhametshin. 2003. "Official and Unofficial Islam." In *Islam in Post-Soviet Russia: Public and Private Faces*, edited by H. Pilkington and G. Yemelianova, 117–164. London: Routledge.

Malashenko, A. V., and A. Nuritova. 2009. "Islam in Russia." *Social Research* 76 (1): 321–358.

Mamdani, M. 2004. *Good Muslim, Bad Muslim: America, the Cold War, and the Roots of Terror*. New York: Three Leaves Press.

McBrien, J. 2017. *From Belonging to Belief: Modern Secularisms and the Construction of Religion in Kyrgyzstan*. Pittsburgh, PA: University of Pittsburgh Press.

Mukhametshin, R. 2010. "Islamic Discourses in the Volga-Urals Region." In *Radical Islam in the Former Soviet Union*, edited by G. Yemelianova, 30–61. London: Routledge. http://public.eblib.com/EBLPublic/PublicView.do?ptiID=465604.

Müller, D. 2017. "'Aber Hocam … ': Imame und die Aushandlung Islamischer Autorität im Alltag von Schweizer Moscheen" ['But Hocam … ': Imams and the negotiation of Islamic authority in the everyday life of Swiss mosques]." *Zeitschrift für Ethnologie* 142 (1): 67–92.

Müller, D. M., and K. Steiner. 2018. "The Bureaucratisation of Islam in Southeast Asia: Transdisciplinary Perspectives." *Journal of Current Southeast Asian Affairs* 37 (1): 3–26.

Rasanayagam, J. 2014. "The Politics of Culture and the Space for Islam: Soviet and Post-Soviet Imaginaries in Uzbekistan." *Central Asian Survey* 33 (1): 1–14. doi:10.1080/02634937.2014.882619.

Rorlich, A.-A. 1986. *The Volga Tatars: A Profile in National Resilience. Studies of Nationalities in the USSR*. Stanford, CA: Hoover Institution Press, Stanford University.

Schielke, S. 2010. "Second Thoughts about the Anthropology of Islam, or How to Make Sense of Grand Schemes in Everyday Life." *ZMO Working Papers* 2: 1–16.

Schiffauer, W. 2006. "Migration and Religion: A Special Relationship." *Fikrun Wa Fann* 83: 29–34.

Scott, J. C. 1996. "State Simplifications: Nature, Space, and People." *Nomos* 38: 42–85.

Stephan, M. 2010. "Education, Youth and Islam: The Growing Popularity of Private Religious Lessons in Dushanbe, Tajikistan." *Central Asian Survey* 29 (4): 469–483. doi:10.1080/02634937.2010.538283.

Stephan, M. 2013. "Duschanbe – Moskau – Kairo: Transnationale religiöse Erziehungspraktiken tadschikischer Familien in der Migration" [Dushanbe - Moscow - Cairo: Transnational religious education practices of Tajik families in migration]. In *Neue Räume, neue Zeiten*, edited by C. Hunner-Kreisel and M. Stephan, 125–140. Wiesbaden: Springer Fachmedien. http://link.springer.com/chapter/10.1007/978-3-531-18948-2_8.

Suleymanova, D. 2015. "Islam as Moral Education: Madrasa Courses and Contestation of the Secular in the Republic of Tatarstan, Russia." *Religion, State and Society* 43 (2): 150–167. doi:10.1080/09637494.2015.1056639.

Yemelianova, G. 1999. "Islam and Nation Building in Tatarstan and Dagestan of the Russian Federation." *Nationalities Papers* 27 (4): 605–629.

Yemelianova, G. 2003. "Islam in Russia: An Historical Perspective." In *Islam in Post-Soviet Russia: Public and Private Faces*, edited by H. Pilkington and G. Yemelianova, 15–60. London ; New York: Routledge.

Traditionalization as a response to state-induced development in rural Tibetan areas of Qinghai, PRC

Jarmila Ptackova

ABSTRACT
The current state-induced and top-down-implemented development and modernization of the predominantly rural areas of western China can be perceived as a clear demonstration of Chinese power in Tibetan areas, resulting in the repression of expressions of minority culture. This article argues that the local population's various practices of traditionalization, as demonstrated through an emphasis on the maintenance or (re)invention of representative cultural forms can be understood as efforts to counteract the socio-economic and cultural assimilation measures or even as a form of political resistance. At the same time, in the context of the economic opportunities brought on by the rapid development, in tourism for example, traditionalization has become an important economic asset for both the state and local Tibetans. These (revived) traditions could enhance cultural awareness among visitors to minority areas and strengthen local people's sense of cultural security and their self-understanding as Tibetans.

Introduction

The state-induced development strategy known as the Great Opening of the West (*xibu da kaifa*), launched in China at the turn of the century (Goodman 2004; Holbig 2004), entrenches the rural Tibetan population more deeply in the general public and administrative systems of China. This strategy not only is visible spatially; it also permeates all of the social and economic structures, as well as traditional habits and values, of minority populations (Yeh 2003; Fischer 2014; Zenz 2014), who are officially labelled 'backward' (*luohou*) (Information Office of the State Council, People's Republic of China, 2015). Minorities' allegedly 'backward' way of life is characterized by an absence of certain material objects in people's daily lives, dependence on the primary economic sectors of agriculture and animal husbandry, and the persistence of local ethnic customs, beliefs and values (Hillman 2003, 86). All this is positioned in contrast to the current Chinese understanding of modernity as defined by the model of the industrialized West (Oakes 1998, 7) and aimed at shaping national consensus and ensuring overall political and macroeconomic stability (Zhao 2010, 423).

Chinese development projects, then, aim to 'civilize' the ethnic-minority populations and wipe out those aspects of their 'traditional cultures' that, in the eyes of the Chinese state, inhibit them from functioning in the modern world (Douglas 2004, 87; Rao and Walton 2004, 10). Even though many of the development measures have been welcomed by the local populations in Tibetan rural areas, the majority of the modernization projects are not presented in a detailed and comprehensive manner to the affected people, and their planning and implementation are beyond their control (Ptackova 2019). For the people, the imposition of such projects often creates a sense of being fully exposed to and dependent upon the governmental management system, and leaves the local populations little space to make decisions about their own lives. This is especially notable in rural areas, where ongoing socio-economic destabilization caused by orchestrated urbanization and the imposition of environmentally conditioned limitations on established livelihoods – measures that are promoted through the Great Opening of the West development strategy – increase the feeling of sociocultural insecurity (Gruschke 2012; Ptackova 2019).

To react to the pressure of development and reach at least a modicum of stability, Tibetan communities have two options: accommodate or resist (Harrell 2001, 24). This entails either adapting as completely as possible to the imposed modernization efforts, or emphasizing the differences between the Tibetan culture and mainstream China's culture and challenging the wave of socio-economic and cultural reforms, aimed at assimilation and unification, that are part and parcel of the politically and economically motivated development initiatives.

While the decision to accommodate is mainly driven by material interests, the decision to resist – that is, to encourage traditionalization and emphasize cultural differences – can be interpreted either as an ideological statement, as a means of maintaining cultural security (Rao and Walton 2004, 15), or as materially motivated, a form of cultural commodification (Cole 2007) whereby recourse to 'local culture and traditions' is used as an economic resource (Comaroff and Comaroff 2009). In the case of the Tibetan minority in China, both decisions can be also strongly politically influenced. Using data collected since 2007 in the course of repeated observations of the social, cultural and economic changes resulting from the extensive infrastructural development and social and economic modernization efforts implemented in the Tibetan pastoral and semi-pastoral communities in Qinghai Province, as well as from interactions with Tibetans living in Xining, the provincial capital, this article provides insight into the social mechanisms and strategies used by the Tibetan population in response to the intensive state development policies. The information presented here stems from formal and informal interviews with rural Tibetans, mostly in Huangnan Tibetan Autonomous Prefecture (Tib.: rMa lho), as well as with Tibetans who had decided to move to smaller or larger urbanized areas of township, county, prefecture or province centres and became engaged in private business or found employment in state service. Huangnan Prefecture is in the south-eastern part of the Qinghai Province and comprises predominantly rural farming, semi-pastoral and pastoral areas inhabited by Tibetans.

During the first phase of the modern development reforms, when economic and infrastructural reforms, following the Reform and Opening (*gaige kaifang*) of the 1980s and 1990s, reached the rural areas of the High Plateau, the vision of socio-economic improvement motivated many Tibetans in Huangnan to choose the trend of modernization. Tibetans were eager to experience the 'taste of modernity', represented by apartment housing, modern vehicles, Western clothing and electronic devices (Iselin 2011). Moreover, these material assets became new symbols of wealth and social status among Tibetans. The socio-economic motivation was thus decisive, and people with the educational or financial means expected to gain higher incomes through engaging in occupations in towns or through businesses connected with development projects. The economic motivation also influenced many Tibetans' decisions concerning their children's education (Grant 2018, 15).

Understanding the advantages and growing importance of fluency in Chinese in the Han-dominated social and economic environment, some of my Tibetan informants[1] in Huangnan who have access to Chinese-language schools in county towns such as Jianzha (Tib.: gCan tsha) and Tongren (Tib.: Reb gong) chose to send their children to these schools instead of the Tibetan-language schools that were prevalent in rural areas in Qinghai (Kolås and Thowsen 2005, 140). Tibetans who moved to the city of Xining, the provincial capital, did not even have a choice in the matter – the capital does not have Tibetan autonomous area status, so it does not have Tibetan schools, and all children must attend schools with Chinese as the language of instruction. Those Tibetans who moved to larger urbanized areas that are dominated by the Chinese population and those who picked new livelihoods targeting Chinese customers or business partners adapted to a Westernized and Chinese-dominated environment. The disconnection from a more traditional way of life in the villages and village communities led to a decline in the practice of local rituals and traditions.

Tibetan intellectuals, themselves generally residing in the city and promoting modernization as the foundation of Tibetan national identity, at least until the early 2000s (Thurston 2018, 154), were among the first to point out the loss of Tibetan culture that was being caused by the overall globalization or 'Sinicization' and exacerbated by the state-induced modernization that the Great Opening of the West represented. The trend of cultural loss and deterioration was especially visible among the children, who were growing up in an increasingly Chinese environment and being influenced by Chinese media. Enrolment in Chinese schools also contributed to a change in Tibetan children's behaviour. After a few years of education, many parents noted, their children were not only learning good Chinese but also adopting the habits of their Han Chinese teachers. After spending the majority of their time in the Chinese-language environment, the preferred language of many of these children became Chinese, even at home. As a result, some of them have trouble understanding, let alone speaking, Tibetan (Postiglione, Jiao, and Li 2014). This was an unexpected outcome for the parents, and led to sociocultural disruptions, especially in rural households, where members of the older generations often have no knowledge of Chinese.

Traditionalization as a response to imposed modernization and induced development

The growing Sinicization, particularly of the young Tibetans who are exposed to the Chinese educational system and entertainment opportunities in the towns and cities, provoked a wave of traditionalization measures that promoted Tibetan 'tradition as a marker of identity' (Beyer and Finke 2019, this issue). Since about 2004 (Robin 2014), the Tibetan identity promoted by Tibetan intellectuals and cultural producers stressed Tibetans' cultural differences in the face of growing Chinese influence on an everyday level (Thurston

2018). In this context, the life of Tibetan herders in the grasslands, seen as representing the strongest contrast to 'Chinese' city life, came to be viewed as epitomizing the 'vision of authentic Tibetan culture' (Kolås and Thowsen 2005, 153). The mass relocation of pastoralists away from the grasslands since the start of the new century and the state's efforts to incorporate them into alternative occupational sectors have thus been perceived by Tibetans as further measures to destroy the core of Tibetan culture and have strengthened the traditionalizing tendencies among various segments of the Tibetan population.

This trend to revive Tibetan traditions has been further supported since 2008, the year of the Olympic Games in Beijing. The international attention to China led to severe unrest in Tibetan areas and encouraged Tibetans to target the increasing Chinese presence. As a result, the central government tightened control in the Tibetan Autonomous Region and other Tibetan areas and introduced new restrictions on minority cultural expression (Leibold 2013). Tibetan traditionalization – that is, Tibetans' (re)invention of tradition to distinguish themselves culturally from the Han majority – thus also needs to be seen in this political context and should be understood as a subtle way of resisting the Chinese state. Although creating Tibetan cultural niches in the Han-dominated urban environment could be understood simply as a form of 'channelling', defined by Grant (2018, 3) as the establishment of ethnic minority spaces by 'customizing of homes, private venues for social gathering, and sites for religious structures and activities', for the Tibetan population in the cities, these niches clearly express affiliation to the Tibetan nationality and feed into a sense of a common (political and cultural) bond (Hobsbawm 1983, 6, 12).

Initiatives to define Tibetan identity through traditionalization and cultural differentiation, or 'Tibetanization' as Zenz (2018) has called it, emphasized the use of the Tibetan language as one of the 'principal markers of Tibetan identity' (Kolås and Thowsen 2005, 14). Dictionaries with invented Tibetan terms for Chinese and English borrowings started to appear in the early 2000s, especially in the eastern Tibetan area of today's Qinghai. Not only intellectuals, but monastic authorities and even members of the rural public started to promote the use of 'pure' Tibetan, meaning without any Chinese terms (Nyima 2017). This presented quite a challenge, as especially for certain terms, including numbers, days of the week, place names and the names of policies, Chinese had long been dominant, particularly in eastern Tibetan areas in Qinghai and Sichuan (Schrempf and Hayes 2010).

Through social media, the new language-purification movement has spread quickly across both urban and rural areas. In Huangnan and elsewhere in Qinghai, people have started to dictate their phone numbers in Tibetan, for example, or compete to guess the original Tibetan place names when travelling. Among intellectuals, associations to protect the mother tongue have been established (Robin 2013). Awareness of Tibetan language use was also strengthened through an emphasis on literature, and new Tibetan-language novels and volumes of poetry appeared in large numbers on the shelves of bookstores. Some of these texts explored themes of everyday life, while others directly addressed the need for cultural preservation, such as poems equating the Tibetan alphabet with Tibetans' blood and body parts (Robin 2013). People paid particular attention to whether singers sang the Tibetan lyrics to songs, especially as state propaganda encouraged people to sing in Chinese even when accompanied by Tibetan music, and many singers complied, to avoid trouble and restrictions. Popular singers can reach even illiterate Tibetans, which makes them a target of state security surveillance and liable to imprisonment for addressing topics such as Tibetan national unity and emphasizing the importance of Tibetan language use. These singers have become icons among the Tibetan public. Besides championing the issue of Tibetan language use, they help promote trends in fashion. By wearing robes or new clothing designs that display features or ornaments that are regarded as 'traditionally Tibetan' but which are made to suit everyday life in the cities, the artists help reintroduce a sense of Tibetan culture and tradition into the daily lives of (young) people, particularly in urban places. Efforts to curb these activities, and other signs of repression such as regular arrests of singers, famous artists and other publicly recognized personages, usually only strengthen Tibetans' sense of loss of control over expressions of their own cultural identity. This in turn leads to further demonstrations of dissatisfaction and in fact does more to enhance traditionalization than to diminish it.

Another important medium for showcasing Tibetan culture is the cinema. Tibetan cinematography is still in its infancy, having been born in the twenty-first century. But it has quickly become one of the most important tools in the struggle to preserve and promote Tibetan culture, as it grapples with fundamental sociocultural topics, documents traditions and customs, and often addresses Tibetans' search for identity inside modern China. The majority of people involved in Tibetan movie-making started as amateurs, filming what are considered 'traditional culture and customs' from their home areas, such as weddings, song contests and religious ceremonies. More and more motion pictures have also begun to appear, which are increasingly reaching an international audience and meeting international standards. Representatives of the Chinese national security system are ambivalent about Tibetan movies. As Tibetan films and directors become known abroad, it becomes more difficult for state authorities to ban the movies or arrest their producers without causing an international commotion – compared, for instance, to arresting Tibetan singers, who are mostly known only to a local audience. Within China, some Tibetan movies have been awarded national prizes and are sometimes even promoted as part of national minority heritage (Young 2018; Asia Society 2010). But the directors do face strict national censorship and have to be extremely cautious in their selection of topics and the handling of the plot (Phillips 2016). In addition to the proliferation of Tibetan movies, some shows, predominantly Chinese movies and soap operas, are being dubbed into Tibetan, and some Tibetan filmmakers and artists have started to produce Tibetan fairy tale films and cartoons to take the place of Chinese-language television programming for children (Thurston 2018).

The trend towards traditionalization among Tibetans is also visible in the selection of schools. Zenz (2017) shows that there has been a statistical increase in students enrolled in Tibetan-medium education. This reflects the socio-economic interests of Tibetans, who have recognized that, at present, they stand a better chance of finding employment in state positions requiring knowledge of Tibetan, for example as teachers or cadres (Zenz 2017). It also shows the general tendency of traditionalization in the politicized Sino-Tibetan context, which emphasizes Chinese and Tibetan cultural differences (Yeh 2002).

Traditionalization is thus not only a cultural but also a political statement. According to my observations in the semi-urban areas of Huangnan, both socio-economic and cultural-political factors entice many parents who had sent their first child to a Chinese school to place their second child in a Tibetan-language school. To make a Tibetan-language education possible for their children, some of my informants residing in the provincial capital are even willing to be separated from their children, sending them to the grandparents in the countryside so they can enrol in a primary school there. In general, Tibetans still acknowledge the importance of being fluent in Chinese, but they see the preservation of their own culture and language as no less fundamental.

The general mood for Tibetanization was demonstrated and further fuelled in 2010, during the attempt to introduce the Qinghai Province Mid- and Long-Term Plan for Educational Reform and Development, which led to a wave of public protests (*The Guardian* 2010). This reform was intended to abolish Tibetan (and other minority languages) as the language of instruction in schools in the autonomous minority areas, making Chinese the language of instruction in all schools (Robin 2013). For the Tibetan regions, this would have limited the use of Tibetan to *Tibetan language* classes, with all other subjects being taught in Chinese. The government presented the plan as a way to improve the chances for Tibetan students to get accepted to elite universities or to get better jobs. Tibetans engaged in the protests saw this it as an attempt to further suppress their culture. After the widespread public outcry, the government decided to shelve the idea of making Chinese the sole language of instruction, at least for the time being.

The search for a cultural common space of belonging (Grant 2018, 5) led to the emergence of White Wednesday (Lhakar), a movement to establish Wednesdays as a fixed day for Tibetans to take a break from their engagement with modernity and consciously show off their ethnic and cultural affiliation. This started among Tibetans in exile and gradually reached the Tibetan population inside China. Even for those engaged in modern, urban or non-Tibetan-related occupations, this day was intended to become 'an island of Tibetanness', a special time when people eat Tibetan food, wear Tibetan attire and speak only Tibetan (Robin 2013; Nyima 2017). The need to maintain a common pool of shared traditions is particularly important for nationalities that do not have effective control over their own legal, territorial and administrative structures, such as Tibetans. The 'Tibetan appearance' in terms of language use, clothing and other visible markers of Tibetan identity is thus an 'important means of establishing solidarity' (Klieger 2002, 6).

Small-scale gatherings such as the White Wednesday meetings were welcomed in Qinghai, where they became a substitute not only for rural summer festivals, which urban Tibetans bound to the city by their occupation could not attend, but also for the annual Tibetan summer gathering in Xining, a huge picnic with music and theatre performances, which was banned for political reasons in 2008. Although the summer gathering was revived later, monitoring of the participants and new organizational regulations were imposed by the provincial government. Moreover, to demonstrate a notion of social normality, Tibetan companies were encouraged to organize the participation of their employees in the summer gathering. All this undermined the authenticity of the event, and the gathering lost popularity among Tibetans. Instead, Tibetan socializing started to take place in new Tibetan-style restaurants established in private apartments specially altered to suit the purpose (Grant 2018).

Practices of traditionalization are not carried out in the same way throughout Tibet, and the degree of participation as well as the actors involved differ from urban or semi-urban areas to the countryside. According to my observations, the call for cultural differentiation comes predominantly from the Tibetan middle class – artists and members of the intelligentsia leading an urban life – and plays much less of a role among the poorer pastoral or farm households. These differences are most likely due to the more acute need for economic security among rural households, which are engaged predominantly in animal husbandry or farming and are not well integrated into the cash economy. Another reason is that the general need for cultural preservation is not as salient in the Tibetan-dominated environment of the villages. Driven by the need for economic security and attracted by the socio-economic possibilities created by state-instigated development, pastoralists and farmers are more likely to view the option of Chinese education for their children and life in a house or apartment in a (semi-)urban area in a positive light.

Boosting the economy through traditionalization

Particularly in the tourist industry, 'tradition' has come to be regarded as an exploitable resource, especially if it concerns 'minority cultures' (Oakes 1998, 47; Yeh and Coggins 2014; Chio 2017; Comaroff and Comaroff 2009), to which more attention has been paid since the Chinese inland tourism boom. The state's attitude to minorities in the context of tourism stands in contrast to the general socio-economic unification efforts of its development policy. Understanding the potential of multiculturalism – that is, the coexistence of many minority groups and their diverse cultural backgrounds within China – as one of the resources in China's west, the state has begun its own campaign of traditionalization. It is investing, for example, in the reconstruction of Buddhist monasteries and the development of new structures and places of interest using ethnic cultural imagery. It has also opened museums of minority culture and begun to support the preservation of traditional costumes, songs, dances and customs (Schrempf and Hayes 2010).

But this state support of ethnic culture as an exploitable resource takes place in a selective manner driven predominantly by the 'politics of appearance' (Chio 2014, 16). Consequently, the state has chosen the most visually attractive expressions of minorities' cultures. This reflects the taste of the majority of tourists, holding the greatest economic potential, rather than the taste of the minority populations. For example, in trying to broaden tourists' access to 'the ethnic culture' of China's minorities, some villages and tourist attractions have been rebuilt and connected to the existing infrastructure; in other places, traditional houses have been reconstructed to be both more 'ethnic' and more comfortable for tourists (Zimmermann 2014; Chio 2017). Elsewhere, local names and legends have been reinvented to suit the visitors' expectations (see e.g. the case of Shangri-la in Hillman 2003). At major tourist sights, not only in Tibetan areas, it is common to encounter members of other ethnic groups dressed in the traditional attire and performing as the promoted minority (see Schlehe and Uike-Bormann 2008 for Southeast Asia). Examples include the Hui businessman adopting a Tibetan identity in Shangri-la, Yunnan (Hillman 2003), and state-employed ethnic Hans dressed as Tibetans in Kumbum, Qinghai, or as Huis in the Park of the Hui Muslim Culture in Ningxia.

It is not always national security reasons that determine the choice of suitable representatives of a particular ethnic group at a tourist site, such as having Han Chinese represent Tibetans in Tibetan monasteries. In some cases, the visual ethnic 'authenticity' expected by tourists plays a role (Oakes 1998, 26; Notar 2006, 66; Kolås 2008, 126). This more 'authentic' image can often be better conveyed by an employee dressed in an ethnic costume than by actual members of the ethnic group who underwent a shorter or longer process of cultural assimilation (Harrell 2001) and who, in their Western suiting, may not appear 'traditional' enough for the expectations of tourists.

The economic exploitability of ethnic culture has not been discovered only by the state and supra-regional tourism companies. Local Tibetans and members of other ethnic groups are also trying to take advantage of their cultural uniqueness to make money through the commodification of their culture (Walsh 2005) or through the authentication of items that are 'inauthentically' produced, that is, in ways that reflect larger global patterns of production (Notar 2006, 66). Traditionalization in this context is thus selective and engages in the conservation of certain marketable cultural aspects of the past (Comaroff and Comaroff 2009, 8–10), or their imitations. An increase in the local GDP through income generated from ethnic tourism is included in the overall development plan for the Tibetan areas in Qinghai, where it is expected to replace the lost income from animal husbandry in those areas where the pastoral population has been relocated (Zeku 2007, 5). But in terms of management, financial means and social and administrative connections, small local initiatives can hardly compete with larger enterprises and the state, which end up with the biggest share (Kolås and Thowsen 2005, 168; Notar 2006).

The promotion of ethnic culture to satisfy tourists rather than to uphold the unique ways of life and customs of minorities is often perceived as a threat to the 'endemic culture' because it reduces culture to colourful costumes, songs, and rather 'primitive' customs and eventually transforms tradition, material culture and (sacred) spaces into commodities (Sutton and Kang 2010, 106; Coggins and Yeh 2014, 5). Yet it also has the potential to establish a 'rural modernity' (Chio 2017, 422) or an 'authentic modernity' (Oakes 1998, 7), allowing locals to combine their ethnic culture with the market economy.

Moreover, promoting ethnic culture in this way raises consciousness not only among members of other Chinese ethnic groups, especially the Han majority (Hillman 2003; Makley 2010), but also among locals themselves. The newly ethnicized cultural sites in the Tibetan areas of Qinghai, for example, designed in the first place to satisfy tourists, have been appropriated by locals for their daily rituals, pilgrimages and other festivities. In Qinghai it is now mainly local Tibetans who circumambulate the bodhisattva statue in the newly decorated square in front of Rebgong monastery in Tongren or the Panchen Lama temple at the top of Happy Mountain in Zeku County (Tib.: rTse khog). The largest prayer wheel in the 'culture park' in Guide County (Tib.: Khri kha) is frequently visited by Tibetans from near and far and is fast becoming one of their pilgrimage destinations. Tibetan-style hotels and gastronomic facilities, such as the Tibetan tent oasis in Yushu (Tib.: Yul shul – see Chies 2018), have become popular locations for casual and festive gatherings of local Tibetans, who even outnumber the tourists.

The support of minority culture to boost tourism does not take place with the same degree of intensity in all minority areas. In Yunnan, for example, the state's support of Buddhism is obvious from the newly built temples, but in the Tibetan autonomous areas in Qinghai, the government in 2017 banned construction of all buildings and facilities connected to religion, including public prayer wheels in residential areas. The differential treatment goes hand in hand with the different national security perceptions of the individual regions. The multi-ethnic province of Yunnan is believed to be politically more stable (Mortensen 2016) than Qinghai, whereas many of the Tibetan autonomous prefectures and counties have been labelled hotspots of (potential) unrest. As a result, in 2017, the year of the 19th National Congress of the Communist Party of China, stricter regulations were imposed on areas such as Qinghai, where the potential for political instability was believed to be higher.

The state's efforts to generate income from tourism also boost the traditionalization of local handicrafts. Vocational training is part of the requalification programmes for the rural population participating in state-planned urbanization projects. Courses in traditional handicrafts such as carpet weaving, stone carving, and the painting of *thangkas* (tapestries depicting religious images) are among the most frequently offered in Tibetan areas in Qinghai. While such vocational training courses might contribute to the preservation of traditional arts and handicrafts, in many places they have proven to be less effective in developing the local economic base. Rural Tibetans who have successfully established livelihoods on the basis of such vocational training are rare (Childs, Goldstein, and Wangdui 2010). Most of the new opportunities associated with these developments are being seized by people from urban areas or those who already have business experience, not by members of the rural Tibetan population (Wang 2008, 134). In most cases, the vocational training becomes exploitable only with the assistance of a third party that acts either as a wholesale buyer of the goods or as a manager of the workers. Examples of this include foreign NGOs and companies running Tibetan carpet weaving or yak cheese production, and the state ordering large quantities of handicrafts to decorate tourist sites. The state-ordered and state-funded carved stone walls in Qinghai's Kanbula Park and at the Hor Monastery in the new settlement of Heri in Qinghai represent another example of the Chinese state promoting a 'traditional' handicraft, in this case, stone carving, as a new source of income (Ptackova 2015).

Under certain circumstances traditionalization can also function as a means of applying political pressure. In contrast to those cases in which the expression of cultural otherness is intended to make Tibetans feel more secure in their culture and identity, sometimes the Chinese state itself enforces ethnic traditions to demonstrate 'social normality'. One such case is the encouragement to participate in the above-mentioned Tibetan summer gathering in Xining. In a similar manner, traditional festivities in Tibetan areas can be enforced by the state if locals decide to cancel them, for example to mourn victims of self-immolation or protest political repression. The state's directive that Tibetan cadres and state employees must wear robes with 'traditional' fur trimmings when attending state-organized festivities such as the Chinese New Year celebrations needs to be seen in this light (French 2007). Wearing the fur of wild animals, originally a symbol of wealth and social status among Tibetans, has been largely abandoned in the Tibetan areas since the Dalai Lama called for wildlife conservation and environmental protection in 2006 (*The Telegraph* 2006). The obedience to the Dalai Lama angered Chinese state authorities, who subsequently tried to counteract the social movement among Tibetans to dispose of their fur accoutrements by mandating that state officials engage in the presumably traditional practice of wearing furs during special events (Yeh 2013).

Modernization – a threat to Tibetan tradition?

Socio-economic development, top-down urbanization and the market economy are often regarded as dangers for some 'authentic' traditions connected to the rural lifestyles of Tibetan pastoralists and farmers (Klieger 2002). With the propagation of new livelihoods, certain emblems of traditional life, such as the heavy, long-sleeved Tibetan robes designed to protect their owners in the cold grasslands, become unnecessary or impractical. Other expressions of traditional customs become impossible. Among these are, for example, incense burning and conch-shell blowing rituals in new apartment buildings. Some traditions vanish (or are transformed) in light of new demands imposed by a cash economy. In the search for (seasonal) employment and the simultaneous abandonment of tilled fields or livestock herds, rural Tibetans are becoming more mobile. This hinders the performance of rituals linked to the village of origin, such as the *labtse* ritual for the local protective deity, in which the male head of each household should take part.

Living according to traditional social rules might also get too expensive. Besides large family rituals at which several monks or even entire monasteries are involved and need to be paid, the expectation to fulfil certain social customs, such as giving money to the children of relatives and friends, can prevent people, especially of the younger generation, from visiting their birth homes too often. The tradition of the eldest son taking care of the parents when they become old and even, if necessary, of his siblings is also becoming costly. Having to provide for one's own household, the household of the parents and eventually for the school or university fees of one's siblings is a heavy financial burden, especially with development-related pressures steadily pushing up costs. Such traditional tasks and practices, which substitute for state social welfare, often cannot be maintained and have to be adjusted to suit the modern environment.

With the social or economic development of any society, especially when people's lives and livelihoods are also changing, what 'tradition' means and how it is practised change as well. However, as this article has shown, even the very rapid and state-supervised modernization processes that we are witnessing in the Tibetan areas of China do not inevitably mean a loss of 'tradition' or 'culture'. They can also lead to a sort of cultural development, even revival, and produce new outcomes in the name of 'tradition' (Kolås and Thowsen 2005, 172). By (re)inventing certain aspects of local tradition and adapting practices that are introduced as 'traditional' to the modern environment, both Tibetans and the Chinese state engage in the creation of 'alternative modernity' (Oakes 1998, 36). This stimulates the 'cultural survival' (Comaroff and Comaroff 2009, 2) of ethnic groups. In this context, the widening market augments rather than hinders cultural transformation; it not only satisfies the Tibetan appetite for Western fashion, household equipment and electronic devices, but also addresses the need to preserve cultural identity and provides goods that are designed in line with or according to what people consider traditional Tibetan fashion and customs (Grant 2018, 22). Under these circumstances, the achievements of modernization can stimulate certain expressions of Tibetanness. Young Tibetans, for example, are rarely seen with manual prayer wheels anymore, and their hectic urban lives, with fixed working days and hours, leave no time to observe all the rituals their parents used to observe. Religious gadgets such as electrically illuminated decorations for household shrines and small electric or solar-driven prayer wheels in people's apartments, offices and cars suit the modern way of life while supporting traditionalization, or rather a neo-traditionalization connected to the expression of religious and cultural affiliation among the young generation of Tibetans. But the most important asset for Tibetans in this period of fast and far-reaching transformation is being able to make their own choices.

Culture and tradition are fluid and prone to change (Beyer and Finke 2019, this issue; Sen 2004, 43; Douglas 2004, 88). It can be argued that this change takes place at the expense of 'authenticity', at least when perceived from the outside. But of greater importance is the perception of the authentic self from the point of view of the actors themselves (Klieger 2002, 2; Yeh 2002, 231). Culture and traditions emerge and vanish, develop and change, according to the lifestyles and preferences of their carriers. As long as Tibetans can draw on the experience of a common history and language to feel secure in their cultural identity (Harrell 2001, 21), whether or not they maintain and display certain visible cultural attributes is not decisive for their cultural consciousness. From this perspective, the vanishing of certain traditions and customs under the influence of such external factors as imposed modernization or globalization represents cultural transformation rather than cultural loss.

It is therefore not the change itself, but the pressure to change and the pressure on the direction of change as exercised in the context of the Chinese state's policies that deflect cultural development and subsequently endanger cultural self-confidence. This can result in an emphasis on traditions as a means of expressing local nationalism, which can eventually come to be seen as a threat to the state's social and political stability (Kolås and Thowsen 2005, 94). In contemporary China, the ability of minorities to influence the changes that are occurring is limited by the top-down design and implementation of policies through orchestrated, large-scale projects such as the relocation and sedentarization schemes that have been implemented in Qinghai under various labels since 2003 and which may be imposed on the entire Tibetan pastoral population (Foggin and Phillips 2013, 1).[2] Uprooting the affected people from their social, economic and cultural environment without offering suitable alternatives can make them dependent on the will and mercy of the state, which provides most of their material supplies, food and cash income. In such cases existential concerns related to physical survival can move to the forefront and displace, or at least compete with, the need to maintain cultural attributes and expressions. When economic and cultural security are jeopardized in this way, people may resort to desperate expressions of resistance, as is illustrated by the many cases of self-immolation in China's Tibetan areas (Woeser 2016).

Conclusion

Because the rural Tibetan population is generally not involved in the planning and implementation of the major development projects that affect them, state-induced modernization initiatives are often perceived as a clear demonstration of Chinese authority repressing local culture. Consequently, traditionalization among Tibetans can be understood as an effort to counteract planned socio-economic and cultural assimilation. In the context of the still very real issue of Tibetan discontent under Chinese administration, traditionalization among the Tibetan population can also be interpreted as a nonviolent sort of political resistance, of 'defining oneself as different from the powerful "Others"' (Klieger 2002; see also Sen 2004, 54). Tibetans assert their different cultural and historical background by wearing Tibetan clothes, paying attention to the use of 'pure' Tibetan language, and favouring Tibetan-language education. The grounds for differentiation between Tibetans and other peoples of China are further strengthened through the administrative division into ethnic groups (Chin.: *minzu*, lit., 'nationalities'), which are inscribed on each person's ID card. This ethnic differentiation not only incites and helps maintain Han Chinese nationalism, but can also encourage expressions of (local) nationalism among the other 55 officially recognized ethnicities in China, further increasing the potential for clashes (Carrico 2017). It also facilitates political surveillance of members of nationalities perceived as potentially volatile, such as Tibetans and Uyghurs, supports the feeling of 'otherness' demonstrated through social, political and economic inequality (Rao and Walton 2004, 16), and contradicts the Chinese state's aim of stimulating sociopolitical harmonization and sociocultural unification through enforced modernization (Ma 2007). On the other hand, officially recognized ethnic diversification has led to affirmative policies for the minorities, such as state subsidies and favourable family planning, education and employment programmes. Moreover, the traditions of China's minorities can be turned into an exploitable economic resource, particularly in the context of tourism, motivating state investments that help preserve or re-establish the various ethnic traditions.

Often perceived as a threat to cultural authenticity from the perspective of an outside observer, economically and politically motivated traditionalization, or perhaps more accurately neo-traditionalization, might from the viewpoint of Tibetans themselves be sensed as cultural empowerment. In this context, we should bear in mind that, in the case of minorities in China, where many aspects of their culture have been exposed to suppression by a regime dominated by others, the continuity and natural progression of culture and traditions were interrupted. Since the liberalization of cultural expressions that started in the period of Reform and Opening in China, traditionalization has helped minority peoples (re)invent some of their forgotten customs and traditions (Kolås and Thowsen 2005, 151, 173), whether for the sake of political control, economic exploitation, or resistance. It is therefore futile to try to distinguish which of the (re)appearing traditions are more 'authentic' than others, as they all hold the potential to strengthen the cultural self-awareness and self-determination of the respective group, at least as long as the people themselves remain involved in the traditionalization process.

Notes

1. Personal names of interviewees used in this article are pseudonyms.
2. Major sedentarization projects implemented since the launch of the Great Opening of the West include Returning Pasturelands to Grasslands (*tuimu huancao gongcheng*), Ecological Resettlement (*shengtai yimin gongcheng*) and Nomadic Settlement (*you mumin dingju gongcheng*) (Ptackova 2019).

Acknowledgements

The material in this article was first presented at ESCAS 2015 in Zürich and further developed during the workshop Practices of Traditionalization at the University of Konstanz in 2017. Further research was kindly supported by the Lumina Quaeruntur programme of the Academy Council of the Czech Academy of Sciences and the programme Power and Strategies of Social and Political Order of the Oriental Institute of the Czech Academy of Sciences. I would like to express my thanks to all the informants who have helped me understand life in the Tibetan areas of China over the years. Further, I am grateful for the valuable comments made by the editors of the special issue, Judith Beyer and Peter Finke, and by Madeleine Reeves, as well as by the anonymous reviewers for *Central Asian Survey*, which allowed me develop this article to its present state. I thank also Brian Donahoe for his patience with the English proof-reading.

Disclosure statement

No potential conflict of interest was reported by the author.

References

Asia Society. 2010. "Pema Tseden: Tibetan Films for Tibetan People." https://asiasociety.org/pema-tseden-tibetan-films-tibetan-people.

Beyer, J., and P. Finke. 2019. "Practices of Traditionalization in Central Asia." *Central Asian Survey* 38 (3): 310–328. doi:10.1080/02634937.2019.1636766

Carrico, K. 2017. *The Great Han*. Oakland: University of California Press.

Chies, M. 2018. "Post-Disaster Development among Yushu Peri-Urban Nomads: Local Agency, Risk Perception and Legal Framework (Qinghai Province, PRC)." *Nomadic Peoples* 22 (2): 222–248. doi:10.3197/np.2018.220204

Childs, G., M. Goldstein, and P. Wangdui. 2010. "An Entrepreneurial Transition? Development and Economic Mobility in Rural Tibet." *Himalaya* 30 (1): 50–62.

Chio, J. 2014. *A Landscape of Travel*. Seattle: University of Washington Press.

Chio, J. 2017. "Rendering Rural Modernity: Spectacle and Power in a Chinese Ethnic Tourism Village." *Critique of Anthropology* 37 (4): 418–439. doi:10.1177/0308275X17735368

Coggins, C., and E. Yeh. 2014. "Producing Shangrilas." In *Mapping Shangrila: Contested Landscapes in the Sino-Tibetan Borderlands*, edited by E. Yeh and C. Coggins, 19–26. Seattle: University of Washington Press.

Cole, S. 2007. "Beyond Authenticity and Commodification." *Annals of Tourism Research* 34 (4): 943–960. doi:10.1016/j.annals.2007.05.004

Comaroff, J., and J. Comaroff. 2009. *Ethnicity*. Chicago: University of Chicago Press.

Douglas, M. 2004. "Traditional Culture: Let's Hear No More About It." In *Culture and Public Action*, edited by V. Rao and M. Walton, 37–58. New Delhi: Pauls Press.

Fischer, A. 2014. *The Disempowered Development of Tibet in China*. Lexington: Plymouth.

Foggin, M. J., and J. Phillips. 2013. "Horizontal Policy Analysis: A Tool to Promote Sustainable Livelihoods Development; with Implications for Ecological Resettlement and Other Major Development Programs in the Tibetan Plateau Region." In *Pastoralism in Contemporary China: Policy and Practice*, edited by Å Kolås and Zhaluo, 3–30. Beijing: Social science academic press.

French, H. 2007. "Tibetans Turn Festival into Mute Protest against China." *New York Times*, August 16. http://www.nytimes.com/2007/08/16/world/asia/16tibet.html.

Goodman, D. 2004. "The Campaign to 'Open up the West': National, Provincial-Level and Local Perspectives." *The China Quarterly* 178: 317–335. doi:10.1017/S0305741004000190

Grant, A. 2018. "Channeling Xining: Tibetan Place-Making in Western China during the Era of Commodity Housing." *Annals of the American Association of Geographers* 108 (5): 1457–1471. doi:10.1080/24694452.2018.1446821

Gruschke, A. 2012. *Nomadische Ressourcennutzung und Existenzsicherung im Umbruch*. Wiesbaden: Reichert.

The Guardian. 2010. "Tibetans Protest against Language Curbs in Chinese Schools", 20 October. https://www.theguardian.com/world/2010/oct/20/tibetans-protest-language-chinese-schools.

Harrell, S. 2001. *Ways of Being Ethnic in Southwest China*. Seattle: University of Washington Press.

Hillman, B. 2003. "Paradise under Construction: Minorities, Myths and Modernity in Northwest Yunnan." *Asian Ethnicity* 4 (2): 175–188. doi:10.1080/14631360301654

Hobsbawm, E. 1983. "Introduction: Inventing Traditions." In *The Invention of Tradition*, edited by E. Hobsbawm and T. Ranger, 1–14. Cambridge: Cambridge University Press.

Holbig, H. 2004. "The Emergence of the Campaign to Open Up the West: Ideological Formation, Central Decision Making and the Role of the Provinces." *The China Quarterly* 178: 335–358. doi:10.1017/S0305741004000207

Information Office of the State Council, People's Republic of China. 2015. *White Papers on Successful Practice of Regional Ethnic Autonomy in Tibet*. Beijing: Foreign language press.

Iselin, L. 2011. "Of Horses and Motorbikes: Negotiating Modernities in Pastoral A mdo, Sichuan Province." *Journal of the International Association of Tibetan Studies* 6: 429–450.

Klieger, C. 2002. "Introduction." In *Tibet, Self, and the Tibetan Diaspora*, edited by C. Klieger, 1–9. Leiden: Brill.

Kolås, Å. 2008. *Tourism and Tibetan Culture in Transition*. London: Routledge.

Kolås, A., and M. Thowsen. 2005. *On the Margins of Tibet*. Seattle: University of Washington Press.
Leibold, J. 2013. *Ethnic Policy in China: Is Reform Inevitable?* Honolulu: East-West Center.
Ma, R. 2007. "A New Perspective in Guiding Ethnic Relations in the Twenty-First Century." *Asian Ethnicity* 8 (3): 199–217. doi:10.1080/14631360701594950
Makley, C. 2010. "Minzu, Market, and the Mandala: National Exhibitionism and Tibetan Buddhist Revival in Post-Mao China." In *Faiths on Display: Religion, Tourism and the Chinese State*, edited by T. Oakes and D. S. Sutton, 127–156. Plymouth: Rowman and Littlefield.
Mortensen, E. 2016. "Prosperity, Identity, Intra-Tibetan Violence, and Harmony in Southeast Tibet: The Case of Gyalthang." In *Ethnic Conflict and Protest in Tibet and Xinjiang*, edited by B. Hillman and G. Tuttle, 201–222. New York: Columbia University Press.
Notar, B. 2006. "Authenticity and Counterfeit Confidence: Outsourcing Souvenirs, Changing Money and Narrating Value in Reform-Era China." *Modern China* 32 (1): 64–98. doi:10.1177/0097700405282348
Nyima, Y. 2017. *How to Understand Growing Awareness of the Need to Protect the Tibetan Language in Tibet?* Chengdu: Sichuan University.
Oakes, T. 1998. *Tourism and Modernity in China*. New York: Routledge.
Phillips, T. 2016. "Tibetan Director 'Injured in Chinese Police Custody'." *The Guardian*, June 29. https://www.theguardian.com/world/2016/jun/29/tibetan-director-injuries-police-custody-china-pema-tseden-hospital-detained-airport.
Postiglione, G., B. Jiao, and X. Li., and Tsamla. 2014. "Popularizing Basic Education in Tibet's Nomadic Regions." In *Minority Education in China*, edited by J. Leibold and Y. Chen, 107–129. Hong Kong: Hong Kong University Press.
Ptackova, J. 2015. "Hor: A Sedentarization Success for Tibetan Pastoralists in Qinghai?" *Nomadic Peoples* 19 (2): 221–240. doi:10.3197/np.2015.190205
Ptackova, J. 2019. *Developing Landscapes and Peoples*. Unpublished manuscript. Oriental Institute of the Czech Academy of Sciences.
Rao, V., and M. Walton. 2004. "Culture and Public Action: Relationality, Equality of Agency, and Development." In *Culture and Public Action*, edited by V. Rao and M. Walton, 37–58. New Delhi: Pauls Press.
Robin, F. 2013. "Streets, Slogans and Screens: New Paradigms for the Defence of the Tibetan Language." In *On the Fringes of the Harmonious Society*, edited by T. Brox and I. Bellér-Hann, 209–234. Copenhagen: Nias.
Robin, F. 2014. "The Increasing Presence of the Disappearing Herder's Black Tent in Tibetan Poetry and Films: Portrait of the Tibetan Artist as a Social Critic." Keynote lecture, Himalayan Studies Conference, New Haven, CT, April 14. http://himalaya.yale.edu/videos/francoise-robin-tibetan-poetry-and-film.
Schlehe, J., M. Uike-Bormann, et al. 2008. "Staging the Past in Cultural Theme Parks: Representations of Self and Other in Asia and Europe." In *Staging the Past: Themed Environments in Transcultural Perspectives*, edited by J. Schlehe, 57–91. Bielefeld: Transcript.
Schrempf, M., and J. Hayes. 2010. "From Temple to Commodity? Tourism in Songpan and the Bon Monasteries of Amdo Shar khog." In 'Bon: The everlasting religion of Tibet. Tibetan Studies in Honour of Professor David L. Snellgrove.' *East and West* (IsIAO) 59:1–4, edited by S. Karmay and D. Rossi, 285–312.
Sen, A. 2004. "How Does Culture Matter?" In *Culture and Public Action*, edited by V. Rao and M. Walton, 37–58. New Delhi: Pauls Press.
Sutton, D. S., and X. Kang. 2010. "Making Tourists and Remaking Locals: Religion, Ethnicity, and Patriotism on Display in Northern Sichuan." In *Faiths on Display: Religion, Tourism and the Chinese State*, edited by T. Oakes and D. S. Sutton, 103–126. Plymouth: Rowman and Littlefield.
The Telegraph. 2006. "Tibetans Clash with Chinese Over Fur Bonfires", 20 February. https://www.telegraph.co.uk/news/worldnews/asia/tibet/1510990/Tibetans-clash-with-Chinese-over-fur-bonfires.html.
Thurston, T. 2018. "On Artistic and Cultural Generations in Northeastern Tibet." *Asian Ethnicity* 19 (2): 143–162. doi:10.1080/14631369.2017.1386542

Walsh, E. R. 2005. "From Nü Guo to Nü'er Guo: Negotiating Desire in the Land of the Mosuo." *Modern China* 31 (4): 448–486. doi:10.1177/0097700405279243

Wang, S. 2008. "The Development of Small and Medium Enterprises in the Tibetan Regions of China." *Zhongguo Zangxue* 1: 134–138.

Woeser, T. 2016. *Tibet on Fire*. London: Verso.

Yeh, E. 2002. "Will the Real Tibetan Please Stand Up!" In *Tibet, Self, and the Tibetan Diaspora*, edited by C. Klieger, 229–254. Leiden: Brill.

Yeh, E. 2003. *Taming Tibetan Landscape: Chinese Development and the Transformation of Agriculture*. Dissertation, University of Michigan.

Yeh, E. 2013. "Blazing Pelts and Burning Passions: Nationalism, Cultural Politics, and Spectacular Decommodification in Tibet." *Journal of Asian Studies* 72 (2): 319–344. doi:10.1017/S0021911812002227

Yeh, E., and C. Coggins. 2014. *Mapping Shangrila: Contested Landscapes in the Sino-Tibetan Borderlands*. Seattle: University of Washington Press.

Young, D. 2018. "Tibetan Director Sonthar Gyal's Psychological Drama Centered around a Religious Pilgrimage Won the Grand Jury and Screenplay Prizes at the Shanghai Film Festival." *Hollywood Reporter*, 29 June. https://www.hollywoodreporter.com/review/ala-changso-1124123.

Zeku xian Sanjiangyuan shengtai yimin huibao cailiao. [Report on the Sanjiangyuan Ecological Resettlement in Zeku County], 7 July 2007. Zeku xian renmin zhengfu.

Zenz, A. 2014. *'Tibetanness' under Threat?* Leiden: Global Oriental.

Zenz, A. 2017. "Mapping Tertiary Graduate Student Trends and Advertised Public Sector Recruitment in the Amdo and Kham Tibetan Regions." In *Mapping Amdo: Dynamics of Change*, edited by J. Ptackova and A. Zenz, 59–92. Prague: Oriental Institute.

Zenz, A. 2018. "Tibetan Education in China: A Systematic Analysis of Current Developments." Unpublished manuscript.

Zhao, S. 2010. "The China Model: Can it Replace the Western Model of Modernization?" *Journal of Contemporary China* 19 (65): 419–436. doi:10.1080/10670561003666061

Zimmermann, A. 2014. "Chinese Cities as Tourist Destinations: Are Development Strategies at Odds with Tourists' Expectations?" *Zhongguo xibu kaifa yanjiu lianheti di 9 jie xueshu nianhui Guian xinqu* [Text collection of the 9th annual conference of the Consortium for Western China Development Studies], 174–176.

Index

Note: *Italic* page numbers refer to figures and page numbers followed by "n" denote endnotes.